MIRACLES IN MY LIFE

Memoirs of Dr Chee Kuan Tsee

MIRACLES IN MY LIFE
Memoirs of Dr Chee Kuan Tsee

Chee Kuan Tsee
Emeritus Consultant Psychiatrist

World Scientific
NEW JERSEY • LONDON • SINGAPORE • BEIJING • SHANGHAI • HONG KONG • TAIPEI • CHENNAI • TOKYO

Published by

World Scientific Publishing Co. Pte. Ltd.
5 Toh Tuck Link, Singapore 596224
USA office: 27 Warren Street, Suite 401-402, Hackensack, NJ 07601
UK office: 57 Shelton Street, Covent Garden, London WC2H 9HE

British Library Cataloguing-in-Publication Data
A catalogue record for this book is available from the British Library.

MIRACLES IN MY LIFE
Memoirs of Dr Chee Kuan Tsee

ISBN 978-981-98-3286-6 (hardcover)
ISBN 978-981-98-3287-3 (paperback)

For any available supplementary material, please visit
https://www.worldscientific.com/worldscibooks/10.1142/14871#t=suppl

Acknowledgements

I owe Dr. Andrew Peh Lai Huat a deep gratitude for the publication of this book. He has been encouraging and inspiring in sourcing a publisher and in matters pertaining to formatting and editing, as well as suggesting the inclusion of some photographs.

The cover picture is a vibrant painting by Andrew. It is rich with spiritual imagery, blending themes of divine promise, hope, peace, security, protection, abundance, growth, vitality and fruitfulness, all of which are elements of a blessed life.

The first section contains some historical developments in Singapore during my lifetime. The second section contains some societal implications accumulated during my working experience. I am solely responsible for any factual errors and misjudgements in opinion.

KTChee
3 January 2026

Contents

Section I

SG50 — SG60 My Story

This section highlights my medical studies and professional career, my marriage, my medical history, and the conversion of my father. It is also interspersed with snapshots of anecdotal experiences of my life and the changes in lifestyle in Singapore and elsewhere.

Miracles in My Life

There are miracles in all our lives. The growth and development of the complex human being from the fusion of a tiny, microscopic ovum and sperm is an unimaginable miracle. In nature, the little seed grows into a plant with flowers and fruits of beauty to behold. We take for granted that we see and hear, smell and taste, talk and walk, remember and think, sleep and wake as we wish, and enjoy relationships and recreations until we lose the ability and capacity to do so. The ability and readiness to love, forgive and give thanks is also a gift of miracles. However, there are times of losses, privations, afflictions, disappointments, regrets, pain, suffering and sorrow when we ask "Why?" and struggle with the meaning and purpose of life.

This little book came from the inspiration of "SG50 My Story". It is about the miracles in my life. This section highlights my medical studies and professional career, my marriage, my medical history, and the conversion of my father. It is also interspersed with snapshots of anecdotal experiences of my life and the changes in lifestyle in Singapore and elsewhere. In Section II, I have also included views on the changing medical landscape and thoughts and reflections on management and governance collated in the course of my work and my experiences and observations on modern development. The current rapid changes in the relentless pursuit of making or breaking for survival in artificial intelligence (AI) and information or disruption technology are noted.

The Chee's (Xu 徐) Family Roots

There is a legend that a certain Xu Fu 徐福 during the Qin Dynasty (BC 221–205) was sent by the emperor Qin Shi Huang 秦始皇 to go east across the ocean to seek the elixir of longevity. He sailed in BC 219 with 3,000 pairs of boys and girls, presumably to Japan, and settled there instead. Apparently, he changed his name to avoid persecution and established a state to become the emperor 神武天皇 and an ancestor of future Japan. The surname Xu 徐 came from the Xu state 徐国 in ancient China.

However, according to the book of genealogy on my family's branch of the Chee (Xu) Clan, our ancestry dates back to 8th century AD in Henan 河南, central China. Probably due to wars, unrest and military campaigns, there was a migration of families down to the South. My paternal grandfather, Xu Shen Hai 徐深海 (11th-generation genealogical name), also better known as Xu Ji Jun 徐季钧 (family or personal name) was one migratory group that settled in the Fujian 福建 province, Min Qing 闽清 county. The dialect spoken is Foochow (Fuzhou 福州), which is the capital of Fujian. He was born in 1857 and became a scholar and a minor mandarin official at the age of 21 during the Qing Dynasty. However, due to the corruption of the government, he left service to become a teacher. Interestingly, he taught for some years at the local Anglo Chinese 英华 Institute.

In 1893, he was invited to be the chief editor of the Chinese newspapers in Penang and Singapore. The best known was 叻报.

Thus, he migrated with his family to Nanyang. He established himself as a Chinese community leader and chaired the Foochow (Fuzhou) Association. He was active in voluntary and charitable work for the welfare of immigrants from Foochow and patriotic activities for China, such as fundraising. While in then-Malaya, he and a relative established a migrant Foochow community in Sibu, Sarawak. Sibu had also been known as the "New Foochow" 新福州 due to the flourishing and dominant Foochow community there, where even the locals spoke Foochow.

My paternal grandfather had two wives. The elder wife bore him a son and three daughters, and the second wife bore him eight sons. In the Chinese tradition, the son from the first wife was the eldest, and my father, Chee Siew Kee 徐士季 (his family or personal name), born in Penang, became the 5th son in the family. They were all privately tutored in classic Chinese. However, most of my uncles and older cousins went for their formal education in the Anglo-Chinese School (ACS), an English-language school in Singapore. The choice might have had something to do with the Anglo-Chinese Institute, probably a missionary set up in Foochow, where my grandfather had taught. Apparently, my father studied for three years only in ACS, i.e., standards 3, 5 and 7, and took the standard 8, Junior Cambridge Certificate examination at that time and passed. He did not sit for the standard 9 Senior Cambridge Certificate and started work soon after that because the family could not afford further studies for him — my grandfather had suffered a stroke and was bedridden for many years before he died in 1936, one year before I was born. His body was brought back to China in a chartered boat for burial in 1937, during the turbulent period of war. It was a big affair with publicity, as he was a well-known figure in the clan and community. My eldest uncle (Xu Boliang), who made the funeral arrangements, was also well respected for his filial piety and kindness as a medical doctor practicing in the People's Clinic at Rochor Road. He was a medical graduate from Raffles College in the old days. My second uncle also graduated in medicine from Edinburgh, and I believe he was supported by his wife's well-to-do family.

My mother, Teo Swee Geok 张瑞玉, studied in Methodist Girls School (MGS), a sister school of ACS. Both my maternal grandparents were Chinese-educated. My maternal grandfather owned a coffee shop like many Foochow people, and my maternal grandmother was the pioneer Christian in the family. As a result, both my parents could be considered bilingual, as my mother could read the Bible in Chinese and my father could read both Western and Chinese novels. Incidentally, both my grandfathers also practiced Chinese medicine. It is therefore not surprising that we have three generations of doctors to date in the Chee families.

I was born in 1937, with my 13th-generation genealogical name as Xu Chuan Fan 徐传藩 and my family/personal name of Chee Kuan Tsee 徐光志. I am the firstborn in my family. A second sibling died in infancy, thus my third brother Boon Kiat 文杰 has since become my second brother. His family genealogical name is Xu Chuan He 徐传荷. However, thereafter, the traditional genealogical naming was lost in practice. I have three more brothers, namely, Eu Lit 有立, Eu Kee 幼季, and Tsu Hian (David) 子贤 and one younger sister Set Chun (Agnes) 淑从, who is the second last. Due to our affiliation with the Anglican Church through my maternal grandmother, my second brother and his family started the tradition of attending St. Andrew's Mission School.

Japanese Occupation

My childhood memories date back to the Japanese invasion of Singapore in 1942, when I was about 5 to 6 years old. We were then living in a rented two-storey terrace house at 115 Tyrwhitt Road. Somehow, we had an air raid shelter built in the living room on the ground floor. It consisted of a wooden ceiling and floor, with walls built with two layers of plank filled with sand in between. I had no idea when, why and how it was built or later dismantled, but the living room floor sank a little because of the weight. I vaguely remembered that we would hide in the dark and stuffy shelter when there were sounds of sirens, flying planes and bombings.

I was told that when the Japanese came to Singapore, my father, in his early 30s then, was called up, like many others, to a meeting place somewhere. He returned home later with a lump on his head because he had been hit with a baton. Apparently, many others never came back and probably perished. My father was lucky to have been released and even resumed working as a civil servant under the new Japanese government. In fact, he had been a civil servant all his life.

Our immediate neighbour was a Japanese administration agent who distributed rationed rice, oil and cigarettes, etc., for purchase on fixed days of the week. Obviously, people like my neighbour also acted as the eyes and ears of the Japanese. So, we were careful of what we said or did.

Our House and Neighbourhood

Our rented terrace house was opposite the Jalan Besar stadium. Between the stadium and the road in front of our row of houses was a playground with swings, see-saws, merry-go-rounds and a covered bandstand, where a police band would perform on occasions. On the right end of the houses next to Petain Road was a basketball court, now occupied by the building of the Foochow Association. On the left end towards Lavender Street was a cowshed with bullock carts and cows occupied by Indian cowherds.

In front of the cowshed, bounded by Tyrwhitt Road, Horne Road and the facing Hamilton Road, was the newly completed Anglican Church, viz. Holy Trinity Church. Services were initially conducted in Foochow and Hokkien 福建 dialects. It has a unique Chinese-style roof with green tiles imported from China. Besides being a place of worship, it was also a place of refuge for members in the early days of the war. Apparently, a Christian Japanese officer visited the church and left us alone. The church was less than a two-minute walk from our house, and we spent much time there participating in its activities. There was a badminton court in the hall downstairs and we played regularly there when we were young. The church has now been gazetted as a heritage building. I have been attending its Foochow vernacular services all these years and singing in the choir since I was 17 years old. English and Mandarin services had been gradually introduced to cater to the younger generations. Due to the bilingual policy, the vernacular congregations have dwindled. Over the years, all my contemporaries have left for other English-speaking churches. However, I am still in touch with James Lau and Mok Choon Hoe, who have been friends for over 60 years. Choon Hoe's home was a 3rd-storey walk up flat along Hamilton Road next to the church. The open rooftop was our favourite haunt. When we were students, we gathered there with others, very often in the evening to snack, yarn and watch the moon and stars in the sky while lying or sitting on foldable canvas beds. Later, we lost track of one another because of our work and families. However, we reconnected in recent years. Now, we meet every few months with our wives for a meal and fellowship, reminiscing about the old days and talking about our faith, blessings from God, and health issues.

Our two-storey terrace house had a wooden staircase and a wooden floor upstairs. There was a long, spacious and open-air courtyard behind on the ground floor. The courtyard was enclosed by the back wall of the house from the long lane outside the row of houses. There was a concrete spiral staircase that joined the courtyard to the back of the upper storey. We would play and keep chickens during the Japanese Occupation. At night, we would catch chickens, put them in a large basket, and lock them up in the bathroom beside the courtyard to prevent any thief from climbing in to steal them, which had previously happened. After the war, we kept two pet dogs in the courtyard. We were so attached to the dogs that when they were put to sleep because of age and infection, we grieved for two weeks. Thereafter, we stopped having another dog as a pet. Next to the backdoor inside the house was the squatting bucket system toilet. The nightsoil worker would come periodically to remove the filled-up bucket from a trap door below the pit opening through the wall facing the back lane and replace it with a clean bucket. There was an established riddle about which vehicle had the most doors. It was, of course, the nightsoil collection truck with rows of compartments storing the buckets. Years later, during our teens, a sewage system was built, and we had a flushing toilet, a squatting type, upstairs and downstairs.

Outside the terrace houses was a broad pedestrian pavement or "five-foot way", where people walked, cycled, gathered and talked. A wide and deep drain ran parallel between the five-foot way and the road. In front of each house, there was a concrete slab connecting the five-foot way and the road over the drain like a "bridge". During heavy rain, the water in the drain would rise to the level of the "bridge" and five-foot way. Big rats could be seen swimming and scampering about. The "bridge" was broad enough for two persons to walk side by side and strong enough for a motorcycle to ride over. Along each side of the road was a metre-wide of grass kerb. Many households converted the little strips of land nearest to them into vegetable patches. We grew spinach with stems the size of a finger and leaves as big as a palm. When boiled, the soup tasted to us like chicken broth!

There was a balcony in front on the upper storey, jutting out over the five-foot way below. In the evening, we would lower a basket tied to a string or rope to buy food, titbits and supper from the hawking vendors downstairs. We would wait for the calls or sounds of their trades. The neighbours would do the same.

During the day, we would play football with small rubber balls on the basketball court or the playground opposite. We would play for hours with anyone available, as school was only half a day. My younger brother and I were solid fullbacks. We were invited to play by the betting teams for them. We played gladly just for pleasure. We also caught colourful fish from the nearby drain and canal and spiders from the bushes for fighting matches. We also played with tops and marbles, which required some practice and skill. Tops were made by a small Javanese community living behind along Petain Road. By mixing with the neighbourhood children, we learnt to speak Malay and Chinese dialects.

The now-defunct New World Amusement Park along Jalan Besar (meaning Big Road in Malay) was a 10-minute walk from our house. Admission in the evening was by a small fee. It provided entertainment and recreation for mostly the local folks around. In the early evenings and nights, the amusement park was brightly and colourfully lit up. It was lively and crowded like a carnival. There were games and stores, little eateries selling drinks and snacks, and the Tai Tong Chinese Restaurant where dinners and receptions were held. Children loved the joy rides, while idling adults would stand and stretch around the periphery of the "getai" for a free show. The "getai" literally meant "song stage". Performing artists would sing popular and evergreen songs, dance simple steps and put up skits for laughs, magicians would perform their tricks, and a small band of half a dozen musicians would provide the backup music. In front of the performing stage were open-air tables and chairs for the paying customers who ate, drank and watched the shows. There were also Chinese "wayangs", or stage shows, performing traditional Chinese operas. When it rained, the shows would be cancelled. In addition, there were two cinemas: the Sun Cinema screened Western and other language movies and the Grand Cinema screened only Chinese movies. They were ventilated by ceiling fans. My father would take the family to movies occasionally when we were young. Later, we would go on our own. I remember watching Tarzan, acted by Johnny Weissmuller, Western cowboy films with John Wayne, and Hong Kong movies.

Besides the New World Amusement Park, there were two other big amusement parks in Singapore. They were Happy World in Geylang Road and Great World in Kim Seng Road. These are no longer around due to urban development.

Sojourn in Cameron Highlands

Not long after the Japanese invasion, for reasons I never knew, I left Singapore with my paternal grandmother and some older cousins by train and then by road to Cameron Highlands. Perhaps it was because I was the eldest, with two younger brothers aged 3 and 4. Or perhaps it was for my own safety, and there would be one less mouth to feed. An uncle had a colonial holiday bungalow in Ringlet. The house was surrounded by fertile farmland.

Cameron Highlands was then apparently a holiday resort for the well-to-do and expatriates. It was green and cool with crisp and fresh air. Beautiful European-style bungalows dotted the hills. The whole area was full of green plants, fruit trees and colourful flowers, especially roses. I became a farm boy doing odds and ends for my older cousins in their late teens. We grew cabbages as big as basins, sweet potatoes as huge as an adult's leg, radishes the size of an arm, and beans. One of my tasks was to look for a special plant to pound its roots with a stone to squeeze out the milky sap. The milky sap was then mixed with water to be sprinkled on the plants and vegetables as an insecticide using frayed, pounded roots as brushes. I also killed crickets hidden in holes with a long stick. At night, we would catch fireflies and put them in a bottle to shine as light.

Our staple diet was simple. We ate sweet potato porridge most of the time, with fried cabbage. A treat would be steaming-hot rice mixed with pork lard, soya sauce and a fresh egg. There was occasional meat. We even ate snake, which tasted like chicken neck. During harvest time, my cousins would carry the farm produce in huge rattan baskets hung on bamboo sticks or poles and sell them in the Ringlet market, some walking distance away. With the money earned, we would buy "baos", or Chinese dumplings, snacks and rice. It was a treat to look forward to.

My fondest memories in Cameron Highlands were those of playing in the stream by the edge of the farm on one side and the mountains on the other. The stream was about 20 feet wide and less than a foot deep. The clean, clear and sparkling water flowed continuously from the mountains over small stones and pebbles. Sometimes we would build a little dam with the stones. Alongside the stream could be found watercress, which we sometimes gathered for cooking. The surroundings were peaceful and cool. On the mountains we could see "sarkais", or the local aboriginals, and their huts. Sometimes we could see them bathing in the open. They used water collected and carried by bamboo cut in half and relayed like pipes from higher up. My most nostalgic memory was seeing the smoke from their cooking rising in the distance.

Back Home

I stayed in Cameron Highlands for less than a year and was "called back". My third brother, Eu Lit, who was about 2–3 years old then, went in my place to Cameron Highlands. He stayed on till liberation. Meanwhile, my fourth brother had arrived. As he was born during the Japanese Occupation, he was nicknamed "Japanese boy", but also called "baby", which later became "Bobby". My second brother, Boon Kiat, and I began learning about babysitting and housekeeping. Our mother was not in good health and was often in and out of hospital. Incidentally, we were all born in Kandang Kerbau Hospital (KKH). I would carry my youngest brother about and feed him. I learned to wash clothes on a serrated wooden board, cook rice, boil water and fry salted fish over a clay stove, burning charcoal or wood. I also learned to sew and patch up holes in the mosquito net, which we used at night.

My father would sometimes bring friends home to play mahjong. They liked to drink "toddy", an alcoholic drink made from fermented coconuts. They would send us on errands with tips. There was a shop opposite the New World Amusement Park selling Indian curry and toddy. The Indian man who served was huge and fierce-looking, bare-bodied, and had a protuberant tummy. On the one hand, it was scary to meet him, but on the other hand, we enjoyed stealing sips of toddy from the containing mug.

When the Japanese lost the war and surrendered, and the British returned in 1945, it was time for me to start attending school. My mother only taught us the alphabet and how to read whatever simple children's books that were available. I still remember reading "Old Lob's Home". So, it was starting from scratch for me when I went to school at about the age of 9 in 1946.

I started school at Anglo-Chinese Continuation School (afternoon session) in Coleman Street, following in the footsteps of family members before me. My sixth uncle, who was single, unemployed and living with us, then volunteered to send me to school and bring me home on the bicycle. However, after a couple of months or so, he found work in Kuala Lumpur and left. I was stranded without transport.

It was out of the school term. Through contact with a cousin teaching, my mother quickly enrolled me into Chong Cheng Primary School 崇正学校, which agreed to accept me. It was at Aliwal Street in the Kampong Glam area, which was not too far from our home. I broke the family tradition of attending ACS and was the first person to study in a Chinese school. There was this "Ah Chek" or uncle who plied me in his trishaw. When he was not available, I would walk. My stay in Cameron Highlands had helped me to be more independent. I did well in school with a double promotion and made friends with classmates of different backgrounds. We studied civics and values in life besides regular subjects. During Monday school assembly, we would sing the Republic of China (ROC) national anthem and bow three times before the large portrait of Dr. Sun Yat-sen 孙中山, the Founder of the ROC, on the wall at the back of the stage. Near the school along North Bridge Road towards Arab Street was a small post office in a row of low two-storey terrace houses characteristic of the period. We were encouraged to save money, and I had a little "stamp" book to stick on special 10 cents worth of "saving stamps". Over a period, dollars were accumulated. That was the beginning of my saving habits and thriftiness.

Chinese Schools of the Past

I completed my primary education in 1950. Being Chinese-educated, I had no alternative but to continue with a Chinese high school. The choice was between Chung Cheng High School and Chinese High School 華侨中学. I was not very clear about the decision to study in Chinese High School at Bukit Timah Road, which was quite far away. I was 13 going on 14 years old, but most of my classmates were older because of the war. A few were 12 years old and perhaps even a year younger. Many of them came from different states of Malaya. I knew of classmates who had to work at the same time, e.g., by distributing newspapers, helping their parents in the laundry business, or hawking stalls before or after school.

The Chinese high schools in Singapore then followed the school system in China. It was a six-year system, viz., three years in Junior middle high followed by three years in Senior middle high. On completion, it would be equivalent to Form 6 of our former system or the Junior College (JC) "A" level system of our current education system, with supposed eligibility for direct entry to a university. At that time, there was no streaming. Everyone studied the same subjects. The subjects included Chinese literature, English language, Mathematics, Physics, Chemistry, Biology, History and Geography. Except for English language, which was taught mostly by local qualified teachers, all the other textbooks were in Chinese, which was also the language of instruction. Out of the six years of history and geography, four years of materials were on China. So, to this day, I am familiar with the dynasties, emperors, sages, scholar officials, provinces and cities and Confucius culture in China.

Most, if not all, of our teachers were graduates from China. They came from different provinces in China and spoke with different accents. They not only taught their subjects but also talked about life. A few had leftist political inclinations. By and large, they were professional and dedicated in their teaching and lived modestly. Our school fee then was $10 a month, which was quite costly at that time because it was not a government school. The Chinese schools then were mainly supported by Chinese businessmen and philanthropists. The Chinese High School was founded by the well-known Mr. Tan Kah Kee.

In the first year, I took the school bus. We had much fun in the bus and would tease the girls of our sister school, the Nanyang Girls School, next door, chanting about love. Subsequently, I travelled by public transport, which was cheaper. I would travel to school and back by bus. First, I took the Singapore Traction Company (STC) bus, which cost 5 cents, half price for students, to Queen Street and then changed to the Green Bus, paying 10 cents all the way to the school gate, and walked up the slope to the classroom. At that time, there were still a few STC trams running on tracks and powered by electricity carried by cables above. There was a conductor in each bus carrying a shoulder bag for fares collected and a small board fixed with different denominations of tickets on it. The strips of tickets had a number of stops on them, and the bus conductor would clip a hole in the ticket, indicating the stop of embarkation. Along the way, the inspector would jump in to make spot checks. Sometimes, my older cousin King Ting, with whom I had been in Cameron Highlands, who was then staying with us, attended the then Malayan University at Bukit Timah Road, would give me lifts on his motorcycle when his study timetable permitted.

I was given $5 a week for bus fares and to buy lunches in the school canteen on three ECA (extra-curricular activity) days a week. There was leftover money if I had not spent it on other things. Out of the remainder of the money saved, I was able to contribute $1.50 a month to a classmate, who came from a poor family and who had just lost his father. Someone in the class had suggested the collection, and several of us rallied to support.

The first four to five years in Chinese High School were peaceful and routine. During this period, I read more English books than Chinese. It was partly due to the influence of my family, who were all educated in English, and partly due to the people in the church. However, the strongest reason was that I wanted to study medicine and be a medical doctor, again due to family influence. This was at the expense of my command and proficiency in the Chinese language. My standard of English was the envy of my classmates, but my Chinese score was below average, though I still passed. I am trying hard not to forget what I had learned.

I read many English classics in their original versions, e.g., *Pride and Prejudice* by Jane Austen, *Wuthering Heights* by Emily Bronte, *Tess of the D'urbervilles* by Thomas Hardy, *Vanity Fair* by William Makepeace Thackeray, *Ivanhoe* by Walter Scott, *The Count of Monte Cristo* and *The Three Musketeers* by Alexandre Dumas, *The Pilgrim's Progress* by John Bunyan, and *A Tale of Two Cities* by Charles Dickens. I also read Western fiction works by Zane Grey, Max Brand, Macleod Raine, Louis L'amour, etc., because my father was an avid fan, though he also read the Chinese classics and books on martial arts. I liked the English classics for their romance and the Westerns because the heroes always won the hearts of the heroines, and the good guys always beat the bad guys. It was anomalous that I read more books in English than in Chinese. However, the Chinese classic *Romance of the Three Kingdoms* was my favourite, even though I respected Lu Xun a lot. I still enjoy and believe in fairy tales!

During the 5th year of studies, i.e., Senior Middle II, there were a lot of fundraising activities for the setting up of Nantah or Nanyang University. Many of our schoolmates, such as Tang Liang Hong, were involved, putting up shows and collecting donations. In fact, the whole Chinese community, from millionaires to hawkers and trishaw riders, contributed. The Chinese-educated at that time had no opportunity for higher studies in Singapore unless they joined the local Teachers Training College or went to Taiwan or China. Those who could afford it perhaps would go to Australia, like Ong Teng Cheong, our former late President, who was one year my senior, and a few of my classmates. Others would go to Taiwan, the USA, Japan, etc. They would study for matriculation before entering universities. But the number was small. They needed to have money and know English. The Chinese-educated considered themselves to be sidelined in opportunities to rise in society unless they had rich families in business. So, politics became important and an issue. In fact, before the moot for the establishment of Nantah, a few of our classmates in Senior Middle I and some other schoolmates, especially those from Malaya, left for Communist China. A few rose up in rank and position later. One of my classmates, Cheam Tat San, who tutored me in mathematics, became a scientist at the Academy of Science in Beijing. I used to send him money, chocolates (which he loved) and scientific books in English when I was working and studying in the United Kingdom (UK). He and his colleagues would translate them into Chinese. As a matter of fact, I was visited by the Criminal Investigation Department (CID) at home one day for an interview. But they knew that I was not politically inclined and left me alone thereafter.

The brewing political discontent and activities heated up and boiled over during my last year in Chinese High School. Classes were disrupted, and activist students took control of the school, calling for meetings as they wished. We did not take part in their activities, and they were unhappy with us and treated us like pariahs. But they knew we were neutral. Initially, we organised ourselves to go to school together in one classmate's pickup and go home together because the gates were manned and monitored by the students. The most frightening news we had was when someone we knew from another class was shot dead in Cairnhill. There were all sorts of rumours about this person and why he was shot.

Later, even other students and perhaps outsiders came to join the activist groups. Ours was an all-boys school, but there were females as well camping in the school grounds. Classes were impossible, and our graduation examinations at the end of the year were around the corner. So just before the last term, we were moved to a government school in the Guillemard Road area. We stayed away from trouble and riots to concentrate on our studies. A few of our schoolmates who were bright became political detainees, e.g., Chia Thye Poh. During this period, I was also preparing myself on my own to sit as a private candidate for the Senior Cambridge School Certificate. I passed my Senior Middle III graduation examinations well and obtained Grade II in the Senior Cambridge School. At that time, the names of all the successful candidates and their grades were published in *The Straits Times*, like the present National Day Awards!

Up till this point, I had never thought or planned on how I was going to study medicine. The University of Singapore did not take in Chinese school graduates directly. However, there had been a special entrance examination for medicine. I missed it by a year, although I knew of a former colleague, Dr. Wong Kum Leng, from Chung Cheng High School, who was brilliant, and made it. He also became a well-known surgeon. I would probably not have made it even if I had had the opportunity to try. If I had wanted to study in Nantah, it could have been by a direct entry. But I wanted to study only medicine.

Studying in an English School

Then, for the first time in history, in 1957, the Government decided to start a class to prepare Chinese School graduates to sit for the Higher School Certificate (HSC). It was equivalent to the current "A" levels system. However, it meant two extra years on top of the six years in the Chinese high schools. It was timely that classes commenced in Beatty Secondary School at Sturdee Road off Jalan Besar, the year after our graduation from Chinese high schools in 1956. The school was a short walking distance from my home. There were about a dozen of us. Three from my own class in Chinese High School, one from Nanyang Girls' High School, and the rest from Catholic High School. Those from Catholic High School were a bunch of brilliant scholars. They had been well coached and prepared by the Catholic missionary brothers. They scored straight As in the Senior Middle III Graduation Examinations as well as in the Senior Cambridge Examinations. They even studied French and scored a distinction.

We were assigned a General Paper specialist teacher from Oxford. He was Mr. Skinner, who spotted a moustache and who inspired us to read, think and discuss widely and in depth. I owed him a lot. We were all in the science class. Beatty Secondary School was an unknown school when compared to other famous schools in Singapore. But from our small class, we produced at least three PhDs for the University, two medical doctors and one pharmacist. Among the same cohort from other classes in the English stream, we produced a High Court Judge (Goh Joon Seng), a pioneer SIA pilot (Low Sin Chock), a lawyer (Anwarul Haq) who was also a state hockey star, a couple of dentists, a founding president of National University of Singapore Alumni Association (Lai Kim Seng) and even a wife (with a PhD) of a very prominent pioneer father of Singapore. Another pharmacist (Koh Kim Seng) from the same cohort obtained his PhD with a dissertation on Myanmar when he was about 70 years old. He had a business in Myanmar. The first President of the reorganised and restructured National University of Singapore (NUS), Dr. Shih Choon Fong, was an alumnus of Beatty Secondary School who came after us.

We sat for the HSC in 1958. We were at least 2–3 years older than our English stream cohort. My results of three principals and one subsidiary were not spectacular. It was sheer providence that I was admitted into the local medical faculty. I knew of others with much better results but who did not qualify. My dream to read medicine came true, and it was a miracle. But I almost did not succeed in doing that.

While waiting for the medical course to start, I worked as a counter clerk at the Singapore General Hospital (SGH), Emergency Department, where the National Cancer Centre stands now. My job was to register patients manually on forms. The place was crowded, noisy and hot, but I knew it was only temporary for me, and besides, I could earn some money.

Medical Course in the University of Singapore

At that time, the medical course was for six years. The first year was premedical, and we had to study physics, chemistry, zoology and botany together with the science students at the Bukit Timah campus. I had to repeat the same subjects in the HSC, although at a higher level. The pace was fast, and much material was covered in one lecture. Soon, the end-of-year examinations came, and I failed botany. A few months later, I failed the supplementary examination again. I had thought that they would not repeat questions on plant taxonomy, but I was wrong. I was devastated, discouraged and depressed. However, I was allowed to repeat the first year, but my bursary of $800 per year was suspended. It was to cover my tuition fee of $600 per annum, with $200 extra for other expenses.

When I repeated my first year, I was already 23 years old. A good friend, David Pung, whom I got to know through the Student Christian Movement (SCM), said these comforting and encouraging words to me: "What is one extra year compared with the many years in your life that you are going to practice." So, I bit the bullet and told myself to be thorough in my studies and not fail again. Indeed, from then on, I cleared every year without any supplementary examinations. Meanwhile, the "super fresh" system kicked in. Students, who were my juniors in school and much younger in age, bypassed the first premedical year (which was eventually scrapped) and became my classmates in my 2nd year (pre-clinical). I was, on average, 5 years older than they were, a complete generation apart. They were all bright and bubbly, carefree and playful. I felt completely alienated and isolated. I kept to myself throughout the rest of the medical course. My only social life was the church and my involvement in the activities of the SCM on the Bukit Timah campus. The SCM was liberal in theology, and

I met and made many friends from Malaya, the other faculties and speakers from abroad. Among our members were the ex-President of Singapore, Dr. Tony Tan Keng Yam, and his wife, Mary Chee. He had been the President of the national SCM. We had regular worship sessions and meetings. I enjoyed the retreats in Malaya, Changi Holiday Camp and offshore islands organised during the vacations. The themes and topics chosen were provocative, controversial and stimulating. Graduate seniors like Drs. Chen Chi Nan and James Supramaniam also invited us to their homes for meetings and meals, especially during Christmas. During the long vacations of the 2nd and 3rd pre-clinical years, I taught English for a few months in Anglican High School, which was a Chinese school in Changi. It was an experience as a teacher. There was no end to marking exercises and examinations.

The Social Medicine and Public Health (SMPH) course during the 4th and 5th years was interesting. We had 10 lectures on philosophy and the Caucasian lecturer would come in a white, short-sleeved shirt, shorts and sandals. Another lecturer, Ivan Polunin, a medical doctor interested in anthropological research, would talk from a chair put on top of the table. Professor Winnie Danaraj, the head of the Department, would bring two of her clerical staff to sit behind the class to take attendance for her lectures. We also spent two weeks on a public health survey, for which we had to submit our reports. My group covered Ama Keng Village. The villagers lived in attap and wooden houses, and some were farmers growing vegetables and rearing pigs and fowls. Wells were still in use, and there was no modern sanitation. We investigated the health hazards and potential sources of infections, e.g., siting of out-house toilets. The villagers were curious and friendly. It was a different perspective of medicine and a holistic education and training.

Many of our professors and teachers were well known for their brilliant minds and skills, but the younger generations of doctors did not know these pioneering "giants", such as Profs. Gordon Ransome, a well-known neurologist; Monteiro, who became an ambassador; Wong Hock Boon, a prolific researcher and a great teacher in paediatrics; Drs. Gwee Ah Leng and Seah Cheng Siang (in internal medicine); Yahya Cohen (in general surgery); and S. S. Ratnam (in obstetrics and gynaecology). Dr. Wong Yip Chong was a "hypomanic" character who would make the whole class laugh from the moment he entered the class to the time he left — his class on psychiatry was always full.

There was a canteen by itself behind the College Building, near the edge overlooking a football field down below, next to Tiong Bahru. It was very popular with generations of medical students who went there for drinks, food and refreshment. The canteen was known as Ah Leng Canteen after the proprietor. Throughout my clinical years, I would eat "bee hoon soup" (thin rice noodle soup) almost every day for lunch. There would be pieces of fish cake, strips of pork, one or two small prawns and a few strands of vegetables. It was served in a large bowl. With the soup, I did not have to order drinks. The meal was affordable and nutritious, and I never got tired of it. If I were thirsty, I would drink some water from the tap. My father worked as a clerk in the Civil Service and was the sole breadwinner. He gave me $50 a month for pocket money and expenses.

We took the final MBBS examinations in February 1966. As usual, medical results always came out the next day after the examinations. My name appeared on the list of successful candidates. One third of the class had to sit for supplementary examinations six months later. I graduated two months short of my 29th birthday. I was more relieved than elated. The year was one year after

Singapore became independent and one year before compulsory national service.

Medical Career

I went for a short break in Malaya to visit some friends and started my housemanship in obstetrics and gynaecology in KKH, where I had been born, under the University Unit (T for Teaching). It was both amusing and a shock when I found out that I had to work on weekends. Work was hectic, fast-paced and tiring. There was rivalry, if not animosity, between the T Unit and two Government Units. As there were only two house officers in the smaller T Unit, my lady colleague and I had to be on call on alternate nights instead of joining the larger common pool of house officers to do one in three calls, which was so in the beginning. Fortunately, this happened during the last month of our posting. This was an introduction to politics at work, even among academics and professionals. Such was human nature. I had wanted to be a surgeon, but my fingers were short, and my palms were sweaty. Putting on fitting gloves was a great struggle and stress.

While in KKH, I bought my first car, which was also the family's first. It was a red secondhand hatchback 850 cc SAAB. It cost $2,500 and ran on a mixture of petrol and diesel, like the motorcycle, and emitted white smoke. But the Swedish "freewheeling" or free cruising technology was advanced. The gears were manual, but there was no rapid deceleration when the foot was off the accelerator, like the other cars then. Now, all automatic cars are like that. The license plate was SN1437. I was told that the number appeared more than a few times in the top prizes of the local lottery 4D. The 4D was and is popular with the local population. It offers hope of winning money and a better life. Gamers are considered foolish and unrealistic. But, in life, hope of whatever nature and however remote a chance is, is very important for people to carry on living. Even those who are well-endowed would need hope of some kind.

After six months in KKH, I joined Medical Unit II in SGH for my second posting. The Unit was headed by Prof. Khoo Oon Teck in internal medicine, but I hardly saw him as he was very busy with many projects. However, I still remember what he had taught, viz., if leptospirosis was suspected, check the urine for bilirubin. The Senior Registrar in charge, Dr. Lim Pin, had just returned from the UK after his scholarship and MRCP. He was full of new ideas and was experimental. He later became the Vice Chancellor of our University. Besides learning how to diagnose and manage diseases, I was also learning more about human nature, such as rank pulling and passing the buck. Hen pecking was the order. But there were also inspiring and helpful mentors.

Housemanship came and went, and I started as a fully registered medical doctor in the Emergency Department (A&E) working as a medical officer. The head was Mr. Gawne, an orthopaedic surgeon from the UK, who was always in a grey bush jacket, shorts and knee-high socks. He allowed us to do many things. Apart from plenty of toilet and suture cases, we also did removal of foreign bodies, applied POPs to fractures, injected haemorrhoids, and performed circumcisions, besides medical emergencies, such as heart attacks and cardiac failure, asthma, and diabetic comas. Saturday nights were the busiest (and worst) when drunkards and casualties of road traffic accidents were brought in by the police and ambulances, especially after the midnight shows. On other days, if we were lucky, we might take turns to catch forty winks in the early hours of the morning. Usually, whenever there was a lull period, one or two of the duty staff would go down to Chinatown nearby to buy supper for everyone. Mr. Gawne was very supportive of our work, and our camaraderie was strong. When we had an off day together, we would go to the beach for a swim and picnic. It was a most enjoyable posting, full of opportunities to learn and do. I was rather good with my hands.

During this period, I read many Penguin and Pelican series of popular psychology, philosophy and theology and the voluminous Clinical Psychiatry by Mayer-Gross, Slater and Roth — I had more or less decided on psychiatry as my career. A main reason was that I have always been self-conscious of my past failure and age, which left a negative impact on my self-esteem throughout my life, particularly in the presence of former classmates and colleagues. Many years later, at a wedding dinner of a colleague's son, I met up with a former Medical Officer who was one year my senior in class but probably 3–4 years younger. I told him I had recently officially retired from service but still continued to work. He was surprised and exclaimed, "But you were my houseman, how could you have retired so early?" I was embarrassed and uncomfortable. That is why in psychiatry, we always explore a patient's past in relation to the present for better understanding and insight.

After completing my stint in Emergency Medicine, I applied to join Woodbridge Hospital (WH) in October 1967 and stayed on without regrets. Not many would have applied for WH in Yio Chu Kang Road by choice in those days. It was far away from the city, isolated and attached with a strong stigma. A posting to WH was like an exile, but its laid-back work routine attracted some who went there to study and prepare themselves for the MRCP examinations. There were more than a thousand patients in WH then, which was manned by 10 medical officers and a handful of senior registrars and consultants, all trained in the UK. We not only looked after the inpatients but also ran more than half a dozen outpatient clinics in the afternoons scattered over the island. We each saw about 40–50 patients in a two-and-a-half-hour session, spending less than 5 minutes on each patient. One of us earned the dubious title of being the "fastest pen" in WH. We also provided consultative services and follow-ups to all the other hospitals. WH was the centre of psychiatry in Singapore until many years later, when psychiatry became important and recognised, and Psychological Medicine Units were set up in the general hospitals.

There was only one fellowship or scholarship awarded each year (or two) for the Diploma in Psychological Medicine (DPM) in the UK. I had to wait for my turn and was selected for the Colombo Plan Fellowship in 1969. The competing colleague for the same Fellowship could not wait and resigned to go into private practice. As a posting in internal medicine was compulsory and an exposure in neurology was desirable, I spent one year in Medical Unit III in SGH in 1970 under Dr. Gwee Ah Leng, who was a renowned physician, a bilingual intellect, and a Chinese gentleman scholar with a special interest in neurology as well as in psychiatry. I learned a lot about life from him. It was a good foundation year for me. I was also inspired by Dr. Fred Jeyaratnam, a consultant physician, later a founder geriatrician, who was fully committed and dedicated to the holistic care of his patients. He was gentle, soft-spoken and patient, and would answer calls anytime at night to come to help. He would sit by the patient and monitor the condition for as long as necessary.

Our New Family Homes

I bought a house when I was still a first-year medical officer in 1968. Somehow, I had always wanted to have a house and a home of my own. It was a two-storey semi-detached house in Loyang South built by the Bukit Sembawang Developers. I was persuaded by a clinical psychologist colleague, Fred Long, to join him. At that time, the house was in the middle of nowhere, surrounded by forests and farms. It was served by the long, narrow-winding Tampines Road through rubber estates and villages. But it cost only $34,000, including the $5,000 deposit (down payment). I was earning only $1,000 a month as a new medical officer, and my father helped me to pay for the deposit. I took a loan with a high interest rate of 8 per cent because I was not eligible for the cheaper Government loan, which required the property to be self-occupied. It was a small but modern house with four bedrooms and three toilets cum baths. The living room and kitchen were very small, if not tiny. The built-in area was about 1,500–1,600 square feet, but the land area was 3,300 square feet. It was rented out when I was away. After I got married and had my own family, we moved in in 1975. It was renovated and extended in 1988, and we have lived in it since, with Fred Long two doors away as a neighbour. Its area used to be surrounded by trees and bushes, a village with vegetable farms, an orchard of fruit trees, a wooden school for village kids, and two fishponds behind our house, which were noisy during weekend fishing. But now, the whole place has been replaced by HDB flats and private apartments. The estate is now served by the Tampines Express Way (TPE), the Pan-Island Express Way (PIE), and even the East Coast Park Express Way (ECP).

In 1970, our family moved to Seletar Hills from Tyrwhitt Road, where we had stayed for some 35 years. But before we moved, our house at Tyrwhitt Road was virtually the headquarters of the Chee Clan. My uncles and families had stayed with us at various times for variable periods when they visited Singapore or while waiting for their own homes to be ready. Our paternal grandmother lived with us till she passed away in the late 1940s. My parents bought a two-storey terrace house for $32,000, which was also built by the Bukit Sembawang Developers. It seemed the Bukit Sembawang Groups was owned by the philanthropist Lee family, and they built affordable houses in outlying places for the ordinary people. Incidentally, when I was in London for my postgraduate studies in 1971–1972, I stayed with my uncle in his Chinese takeaway food shop in East End and did not have to spend on expensive board and lodging. The exchange rate then was about eight Singapore dollars to one sterling pound. I managed to save quite a bit of money and paid off my loan on the house after I returned to Singapore.

My mother was a full-time super housewife and super mum. Besides all the housework, she could cook delicious meals from whatever ingredients were available. She sewed our shirts and shorts when we were young and even neck ties for the Chinese New Year. She was also a DIY person who repaired appliances like the iron, kettle and a dripping tap. She also improvised and recycled utensils. Everything could be of use to her, and so she did not waste. She also invested whatever she had saved in a "tontine" — a "loan fund" popular with housewives then. A group would be formed, and each member would contribute a fixed sum of money to the common pool regularly. A leader or head would be appointed to hold the purse and keep the accounts. Usually, someone would be in urgent need of money. She would apply for a sum but had to pay interest to the rest of the members. If more than one applied, they would have to bid and pay a higher interest rate. Sometimes, a dishonest head or leader would run away with the money. My mother might also have been a mini money lender. She not only made sure that I had enough to complete my university studies but also sent my 4th brother, the "Japanese boy", to study engineering at the University of Malaya in Kuala Lumpur. She also supported my youngest brother, David, born after the Japanese Occupation, to study Chinese philosophy at the Taiwan National University. He, too, went to a Chinese school, viz. Maris Stella Catholic School. He later became an Anglican priest. In fact, Mum was responsible for all our education plans.

However, my 2nd brother, Boon Kiat, started work after his Senior Cambridge and studied part-time at Singapore Polytechnic. My 3rd brother, Eu Lit, started work straight after his Senior Cambridge. My only sister, Agnes, also born after the Japanese Occupation, started teaching after completing her secondary school and contributed financially to the family. Years later, she was awarded a half scholarship to study for a degree in the UK. My mother was also a great believer that sleep was important for intelligence. So, when we were young, she would order us to take an afternoon nap after lunch. She would cane anyone who did not obey. We had talked among ourselves that if Mum had had the opportunity for higher studies, she would certainly have become someone of prominence. My father was, however, rather laid back. He just brought home his pay for my mother to manage. His hobbies were to play mahjong and go horse racing. In his spare time, he read Western cowboy novels and Chinese classics and martial arts stories. When he was younger, he played the mandolin, which I inherited. He was very intelligent and capable and somewhat critical of incompetence at his place of work. As he was not a "yes" man to superiors, he was not promoted till late in his career. He was appointed Chief Clerk not long before his retirement and enjoyed the benefits of first-class medical treatment for the rest of his life.

Overseas Fellowship

My fellowship to London under the Colombo Plan was for two years. I went to London in April 1971 to start my studies and training in the famous Institute of Psychiatry (IOP), University of London and Maudsley Hospital. The people there did research, wrote papers and published books internationally. It is now known as the Institute of Psychiatry, Psychology and Neurology.

As a matter of fact, it was not my first trip to London. In 1968/1969, I escorted a British engineer working for Singapore Airlines (SIA) to London. He was suffering from Korsakoff syndrome, a complication of his alcoholism. He exhibited characteristic memory deficit and confabulation. Fortunately, he was small-built and not too disturbed or troublesome. The flight was smooth and peaceful with two stops along the way. In London, after I had handed him over to the medical staff at the airport, my long-lost uncle Kim, my mother's younger brother, picked me up. It was a happy reunion after many years. He had been a seaman and settled in London. I was to stay with him again during my study and training in the IOP and helped to serve customers in his takeaway Chinese food shop during my spare time. My uncle was an entrepreneur who later started his own ready-to-eat frozen Chinese meals business. He experimented with his recipe and method of preparation and preservation in his kitchen without formal schooling. A few years later, he sold his business to a franchise and retired to Torquay, in Devon, near the sea. He loved sailing.

During this first trip, I took a train from London to Dover and from there a ferry to Calais and then continued by train all the way to Rome, where I flew home. Travelling for the first time on my own, I felt like a refugee on the run and could hardly remember anything. In a German town at night, people observed the traffic light, even when the street was empty. On my way to Rome, I shared a cabin with some Italians, who were noisy and talkative throughout the night.

April 1971 in London was still cold. I was not quite used to wearing so much warm clothing clumsily. These were made in China and bought in Singapore. The IOP was in Denmark Hill at Camberwell Green, which was quite far away from Stepney Green in East London, where my uncle's shop was. I had to take a bus to change to another bus at Elephant and Castle. In the IOP, foreign students like me were attached to the "firms" of consultants as clinical assistants. The local full-time trainees were all MRCP holders. They trained for three years for the MPhil course. My supervisor was Jim Birley, who was also the Dean then. He was a co-author on the research of High Expressed Emotion (High EE). The ward round was multidisciplinary in approach, and everyone called one another by their first name regardless of rank or station. It was something new to our cultural hierarchy and protocol. The schizophrenic patients were encouraged and supported to stay on their own, away from their families. It was another cultural difference, where we emphasise family support and living together. I was somewhat puzzled and disturbed then on how to apply this back home, but now, with changes to our family structure towards a nuclear family, we may be moving in that direction. We saw only a few patients a day and had more time to discuss management in scope and depth. There was also much stimulation from research activities. Lectures were the run-of-the-mill kind for clinical assistants like us, and I frequently skipped the evening ones, especially during wintertime when the days got dark by 3–4 pm or so. Interestingly, the long-stay patients in Maudsley Hospital were entitled to go away on paid holidays during the summer.

At the IOP, we were in regular contact with the "who and who" in psychiatry. There were Profs. Felix Post of Old Age Psychiatry, Lishman of Organic Psychiatry, Douglas Bennet of Rehabilitation Psychiatry, Julian Leff of Social Psychiatry, Michael Rutter of Child Psychiatry, Peter Scott and Gunn of Forensic Psychiatry, Kendell of Mood Disorders, Wing of Present State Examination (PSE), to name a few, Marsden in Neurology, Eysenck in Psychology, etc. Although I was under Dr. Peter Scott for only a few weeks, I gained a lot of useful knowledge and skills from him. Among my contemporaries who later became "who and who" themselves were Drs. Anthony Clare, Maria Ron, Steven Hirsh, Paul Mullen and Ian Brockington, etc. Of all the foreign students, the Africans were the most confident, vocal and articulate. They would discuss freely and argue intelligently. There were others who were easy-going and enjoyed themselves. The consultants did not hold our hands and teach or spoon-feed us. We had to learn by listening and observing what they said and did and pick up what was important and useful. What I found most useful was having the time to read and think. I spent much time in the library in the basement, which was quiet, and I could sit by the open window to let in fresh air. I did not like the central heating, which made me drowsy.

Socially, when we were invited by the consultants to lunch at the hospital canteen, we had to pay for our own. However, the British Council, which sponsored us, would organise fully paid tours for all the foreign-sponsored students to places of cultural interest or short stays in different parts of the UK. I enjoyed the music festival, Eisteddfod in Bangor, Wales, when choirs from all over performed and competed. Wales is beautiful and charming with nice people. I learned to eat Danish Blue cheese and prunes in porridge for the first time. On my own, apart from the standard sightseeing, England, Scotland, Wales and Ireland are truly beautiful and scenic. There was no language problem, except that I had to get used to the different accents. I attended operas, plays and stage shows. Sometimes, the hospital received free tickets for distribution to its staff. A dental friend, Dr. Kwong Kok Leong, would invite me for drives to the countryside and coastal towns like Brighton and Canterbury. The Student Counsellor of the Singapore Embassy also invited Singaporean students for meetings and meals in his home in Golders Green, an upmarket district in the north of London. Incidentally, he was David Pung, the one who had encouraged me to repeat my premedical first year. We had become good friends. He had a charming and hospitable wife, Esther, who was a graduate from the Trinity Theological College in Singapore and steeped in Chinese traditions. He retired from Government service many years ago and passed away in 2012 while I was still practicing psychiatry. What he had said to me at the beginning turned out to be correct. During my free time, I would go down to Oxford Street to window shop. I spent much time browsing in Marks and Spencer and the supermarkets. The Jewish beef sandwiches in Selfridges were excellent. I bought gifts for folks back home. I am still wearing a shirt I bought at that time. Occasionally, I would meet people from Singapore on the streets whom I had not seen for years. During my second year in London, a few colleagues, e.g., Drs. Fong Yeng Hoi, Kok Lee Peng, Lim Hsin Loh, etc., from Singapore also came over to train in psychiatry, and we met socially.

Nevertheless, I was preoccupied with quickly passing my examinations and going home. I was homesick, especially in the early part, and was concerned about my mother, who was afflicted with pain from arthritis of her hips and thyrotoxicosis, which later became hypothyroid after radioiodine treatment.

Coming back to my time in the IOP, I successfully completed my DPM in November 1971. It was mission accomplished. But I still had one year on my hand. The Royal College of Psychiatrists was then not long established. It had commenced conducting the higher qualification examinations for membership of the Royal College of Psychiatrists, viz. MRCPsych to be on par with the other Royal Colleges, e.g., internal medicine and surgery. My DPM allowed me some exemption for the MRCPsych, but I had to wait to qualify for the second batch conducted in November 1972. So, it was back to more studies. I was the first one back home to sit for the new MRCPsych. I managed to clear it on my first attempt. Although I had not completed my two-year fellowship, I was called to return to Singapore in December 1972 because of manpower needs. I was promoted to Senior Registrar as a specialist in psychiatry, a position between the medical officer and consultant. Back home, in appreciation of the sponsorship to the IOP, I bought a new British-made car. The Morris Marina was manual, bulky and underpowered, but spacious.

Union of Two Cities and Families

After obtaining the DPM and before taking the MRCPsych, someone whom I was close to during my HSC days wrote to ask me to arrange for a European Tour on her behalf. I went along, though not as a pair, and joined her in the Cosmos Tour. In the group was a Hong Kong girl. She was petite, pretty, well-groomed, vivacious and friendly. I was strongly attracted to her. I managed to get her contact number and address. I had been lonely and in low spirits despite my success in my examinations and career. In fact, I had been actively looking for a life partner, but because of my hang-ups, I was introspective, introverted, awkward and slow in my efforts. I did manage a few dates, but it was mostly a one-off affair. It was a case of "those I liked, did not like me, or those who liked me, but I did not like them". But a Hong Kong girl was far away from my mind. As a matter of fact, my family and I disliked Hong Kong people. To many, they might be sophisticated and fashionable, but we considered them to be snobbish, pretentious, vain, materialistic and money-minded. A great deal of these impressions came from the Hong Kong movies we had watched. I tried to date her after the tour, but she went to Wales to stay with her friend, an Irish senior district nurse. (This Irish nurse, Bridie Logan, later became the godmother to my son.) There was no further contact after this, and she went home to Hong Kong. Some months later, an Indonesian colleague, Dr. Tanzil, also on Fellowship at the IOP, whom I had befriended, invited me to join his family to tour parts of England. We went to the Lake District and other counties. On our way back, we passed Stratford-on-Avon, Shakespeare's birthplace and visited Anne Hathaway's cottage. I bought a picture postcard and, on the spur of the moment, sent it to her in Hong Kong. Surprisingly, she replied, and we started to correspond. Later, she revealed that she had bought the same postcard when in Stratford-on-Avon. She had graduated from Hong Kong University (HKU) and was working as a civil servant. We continued to write back and forth after my return to Singapore. We discussed more and more personal matters. Her name is Kiter, a Christian name given to her by her aunt Sabrina, a nurse and colleague of Bridie Logan when she was training and working in Wales. Kiter's Chinese birth name is Lee Hang Fun 李杏芬.

After working for a while back in WH, I decided in early 1973 to join a tour to Taiwan to visit my youngest brother, but I was also intending to visit Kiter in Hong Kong. When I first touched down in Taiwan, I was overwhelmed with this feeling of having come home. The people there spoke Mandarin and Taiwanese (or Hokkien, as it is known to us). Chinese characters and signboards were everywhere. There was a strange sense of familiarity and belonging. I was transported back to the experience of my Chinese school days. Strangely, I did not have this feeling and sense when I visited Mainland China later in 1977 with the Singapore Medical Association.

On my way back to Singapore from Taiwan, I transited in Hong Kong to meet up with Kiter. She came to meet me and took me out to a posh hotel in Repulse Bay for a steak lunch. I was touched by her hospitality and kindness. We spent a couple of days together sightseeing and getting to know each other better. On the day I returned to Singapore, she came to the hotel to give me a short book, "Sea Gull", to read on my way home. She has always been thoughtful of others.

Thereafter, we wrote to each other almost every day. We wrote on airmail letters, which were economical and convenient because there was no need to find envelopes and stick stamps on them. There was no short message service (SMS) and no e-mails then, let alone Facebook, blogs, Twitter and Skype. A telephone call cost $5 a minute! I waited for the postman daily. We continued for months, sharing our thoughts, feelings and aspirations. We were open with and close to each other.

Then, I decided to visit her again in Hong Kong and take her to Taiwan for our first official date. We were quite certain about our relationship and feelings, but it was not an exactly happy trip because we were pondering on the pros and cons of being together, especially on her part. She had struggled all her life to reach where she was. Her father had passed away when she was young, and her family was poor, and she had several siblings. She had to give tuition when she was in school and gave whatever she earned to her mother. She was also very active in the church. Her family was Roman Catholic by faith. After completing secondary school, she took up teaching to support the family. However, she was ambitious and studied for matriculation to HKU. It was fortuitous in that particular year, due to unrest, emigration and low enrollment, she secured a place in HKU. By nature, she was active, sociable, industrious and gutsy. She was also always well-groomed and attractive. She not only managed to graduate with honours but also enjoyed the university life, making many friends. The Hong Kong civil service job was prestigious and enjoyed generous terms of employment. She had a bright future and a comfortable life before her. Besides, she had many eligible and well-to-do suitors. So, marrying me meant giving up her job and leaving her family, friends, a promising career, and everything she had lived for in Hong Kong. She knew and accepted that it would not be the other way round, that I should go to Hong Kong. Though I was grateful that she eventually married me, I also felt sad that she had to make great sacrifices. I dared not ask how her mother felt, but Kiter only said that her mother told her to make sure that I was not a divorcee, as I was 9 years her senior. Her mother had been a pious, family-oriented and long-suffering woman. Some years later, she migrated to Toronto, where the elderly are well looked after by the state. Kiter would visit her, her brother, and her sister there yearly. I went along sometimes.

Somehow, I did not formally propose to her, thus there was no proposal for her to accept — such was the mutual understanding and trust between us. We just assumed that we were getting married and went ahead preparing for it. My three younger brothers had married before me and had raised their own families. There was no reason for me to hesitate and delay. My youngest brother, David, in Taiwan, was the first family member to meet her and was happy for us. He reported her in glowing terms to the family. She came to Singapore at the end of 1973 to be engaged in our Anglican Holy Trinity Church, officiated by the Revd. Lai Wen Kwang 赖文光. During the short stay, I tried to introduce Kiter to as many friends as possible so that she would not feel isolated.

In April 1974, my parents went with me to Hong Kong for my wedding. Kiter made all the arrangements. She booked the church and hotel, ordered the banquet, sent out invitations, arranged for the bridal car and photo shoots, and even sewed her own red velvet evening gown for the reception dinner. Her only instruction to me was to wear a tuxedo, i.e., a white coat and black pants with a white shirt and black bow-tie, which was to be a wedding gift from her to me. I had not known what a tuxedo was, let alone own one. But I did as requested. It was a touch of Hong Kong for me.

On 14 April 1974, our marriage was solemnised in St. Theresa Church by Father Martinelli, who had been Kiter's religious guardian and a mentor to the family. The church was more than half-filled with Kiter's friends and relatives. My youngest brother, David, came over from Taiwan to be my best man and attend to our parents later. Kiter was given a one-year no-pay leave by her employer in case she decided to return to work. It was a sensible safeguard. On the 4th day, after our wedding, we went to Europe for our honeymoon.

We first went to London and then Copenhagen, where I attended a 3-week course in Psychopharmacology under the auspices of the World Health Organisation. The participants from different countries were senior and serious people. We learned about conducting research on clinical drug trials in a suburban area away from distractions. I was temporarily separated from my wife, who "squatted" with a friend's friend in the city, but we met when we could on occasion. In Copenhagen, we visited Hamlet Castle, famous from Shakespeare's play. We saw the Little Maid, which was dwarfed by our Merlion in Singapore. The Tivoli Garden was not very impressive. In a little art museum, we saw Mao Ze Dong's 毛泽东 portraits side by side with pictures of Marilyn Monroe. We were wondering what the hidden message was — this would probably have been sacrilegious in China. From Copenhagen, we flew to Amsterdam separately. Due to a miscommunication, we missed each other at the airport. There were no such things as mobile phones then. It took us some time to go around to find each other. When we tried to check into a hotel late in the evening, the counter staff demanded proof of our relationship. We were given a room eventually after he inspected the wedding date inscribed on the inner aspect of our wedding rings. It was laughable that such a thing could have happened in Amsterdam, a city later known for its liberal promiscuity. We went to Keukenhof Garden in the Netherlands specifically to see the tulips, which were in season. Kiter loves flowers. There were spreads and spreads of tulips of various colours and hues in full bloom, besides other beautiful flowers. There was also a brass band marching and playing music.

While in the Netherlands, we visited Biem Lap and his Chinese wife, whom we befriended in Singapore. Biem is a Dutchman, a leftist critical of the Government working in Singapore, and his wife was a Catholic nun novice studying in the National University of Singapore (NUS). They met at the university, and she gave up her religious vocation to marry him. They were both subsequently banned from Singapore and could only meet friends in Johore Bahru. We have lost contact since.

After the Netherlands, we went back to London, where we booked a tour to Land's End in Cornwall. Kiter did all the arrangements. It was a rustic place not often visited by tourists, but there were unusual and attractive souvenirs, such as lights made from sea urchin shells.

When we returned to Singapore, we stayed with my parents in the family house for the first year. We had another wedding dinner for relatives, friends and colleagues. However, it was tough for Kiter to adjust to a new life in Singapore when she had been so independent and active in Hong Kong. She felt isolated and lonely without her family and friends around. She made a trip back to Hong Kong when she was expecting. Our son, Sung Ping 颂平 ("Praising Peace"), was born three days before our first wedding anniversary. Bridie Logan came all the way from Wales for Sung Ping's christening and gave him the Christian name of Damian, a saint of doctors apparently. We later also visited her a few times in Newport, Wales. When Sung Ping was a month old, we moved to our own house in Loyang. We managed to find a maid, and Kiter went to teach in a mission school, Marymount Convent. Her teaching certificate from Hong Kong before her university days was recognised in Singapore. However, our daughter, Yung En 咏恩 ("Singing Grace"), came 14 months after her brother. Life was very tough for us the first few years, more so for Kiter. She decided to stop work for some three years to look after our young children. When they were bigger, Kiter resumed teaching in a government school. It was a blessing in disguise because she was able to later retire with a pension and medical benefits on her own and not be dependent on me. After she had retired from teaching, she worked as a part-time school counsellor for several years. She communicated and connected well with both students and teachers. They are still in touch with her to this day after she retired from her counselling job recently.

In many ways, Kiter is like my mother. She is very capable, super-efficient, creative and a multitasker. She is also the decision maker in the family. She is sociable and outgoing and has more friends than I do. All my friends are known to her and know her. She has always been well-groomed and elegant but inexpensively dressed. She likes to decorate the house, cook new dishes, and organise functions and celebrations for friends and colleagues at home. She loves gardening and has green fingers. Like my mother, she is good at financial management.

Kiter enrolled both our children in Catholic mission schools. Our son, Sung Ping, started school in Maris Stella (MS), a Chinese school, and later attended Victoria Junior College (VJC). We were called up twice by the teachers for his problems. He was too talkative in class in MS and did poorly in his first year in VJC. However, he passed all the crucial examinations. He loved military life and flying. During national service (NS), he was hospitalised for two weeks with a fever of unknown cause, but he insisted on going to Taiwan for his training the day after his discharge from the hospital, so that he would not miss his Officer Cadet School (OCS) course. He completed his full-time national service as an officer with the rank of Second Lieutenant. He qualified for a place in Mechanical Engineering and Architecture at NUS, but at the last moment, decided to read medicine. In the end, he graduated in medicine with an MBBS from the University of London and completed his housemanship in the UK National Health Service (NHS). Then, he did a roundabout turn to join the Republic of Singapore Air

Force (RSAF) as a transport pilot. He was the only medical graduate among the pilots. However, he lost six years of seniority in the SAF because he joined after his medical studies. He read many books on military topics, e.g., wars and battles, weapons and espionage, but he also read widely on serious topics like economics, politics, life sciences, current discoveries and trends. He is now a full Colonel and a commanding officer in the RSAF. Our daughter, Yung En, had no problems in school. She attended Convent of the Holy Infant Schools (CHIJ, Katong) and Temasek Junior College (TJC). She was completely self-motivated in her studies. She was a "Green" person and, during her JC days, even won a Shell prize to a camp in Brunei with her essay on protecting the environment. Perhaps that was the reason why she decided to study in Australia. She did some research on her own and applied for a place in the Australian National University (ANU) in Canberra because there were many Nobel Laureates among the staff. She graduated with First Class Honours with a Star, a rare achievement. From ANU, she went on to complete her PhD at Melbourne University. She is an environmentalist and prefers to live and work as a research scientist in Australia. As a matter of fact, every time she comes home from Australia to visit, she is upset to see a part of nature in our area disappear and being replaced by buildings and roads. We had travelled quite a bit as a family when Sung Ping and Yung En were young. We visited both the east and west coast of Canada and the USA, Europe, Australia, Japan, Taiwan and Asean countries.

Between 2001 and 2002, Yung En manifested symptoms of congenital hip dysplasia. She was pursuing her PhD then and was incapacitated by painful hips. As usual, she surfed the Internet on her own and decided to have the hip surgery in Berne, Switzerland. We went there twice and stayed for two weeks each time. Somehow, we managed financially, even though Switzerland had been reputed to be an expensive place with a high cost of living. But we enjoyed the beautiful, cool, clean and well-organised country. We sailed on the lakes and went up Jungfrau. The transport system of buses, ferries and trains was amazingly integrated and convenient.

Back in Melbourne later, Yung En had another hip operation to correct a failure of the earlier surgery. Total hip replacement surgery was in its infancy in Singapore then. It was unavailable when my mother needed one in the 1970s. She eventually had one side done in her old age.

Professional Horizons and Milestones

In 1977, I joined the second batch of the Singapore Medical Association Tour to China, led by Drs. Colin Marcus and Arthur Lim. It was after the downfall of the Gang of Four and the end of the Cultural Revolution. China was not open to tourists yet. We flew into Guangzhou, where local shops had earthen or cemented floors. From there we flew into Guilin in a Russian propeller plane, which was hot, noisy and scary. But Guilin was tranquil and scenic. After an overnight rest, we flew on to Beijing in a British Trident, which was comfortable. We arrived in Beijing late at night. The door of the hotel was shut. It was dim and quiet inside, and there was no service available, but the staff woke up and prepared a simple meal for us. We were privileged to visit and see firsthand behind the Bamboo Curtain. As I have mentioned earlier, I did not experience the same feeling and sense of having come home and belonging as in Taiwan. We were accorded VIP treatment everywhere. People were serious and cautious, kept at a distance, and looked at us with curiosity. All the hospitals, schools, factories, communes and other facilities we visited were headed by Communist Party Cadres, some of whom were relatively young, not unlike the CEOs of today. The other staff and professionals kept behind the scenes humbly. People everywhere were dressed in plain colours of blue, grey or brown, unless they were military personnel in green. This applied to both males and females. There were few cars, and bicycles were the main means of transport. I managed to catch up with my old classmate, Cheam Tat San, after more than 20 years, though we had kept in touch all the while. He had wanted a bicycle but had no means of securing one. So, I bought a new bicycle and some cigarettes from the Friendship Store, which was open only to Foreigners and overseas Chinese, and rode it out from the shop to where he was waiting. The Friendship Store was stocked with goods and items considered luxurious to the local population. The local citizens were issued coupons to purchase basic needs from neighbouring shops within the vicinity of where they lived. Their mobility to other districts was completely restricted. From Beijing, we went by train to Nanjing, where we visited Sun Yat Sen's 孙中山 mausoleum and the brand-new double-decker bridge across the Yangtze or Chang Jiang River. It was a showpiece of pride built by the Chinese themselves. Today, they have caught up in development and sophistication in a short span of some 40 years after Deng Xiao Ping's 邓小平 open-door policy. From Nanjing, we travelled by train to Shanghai and stayed in a VIP hotel. Here, we saw the first woman with permed hair. During the whole tour, we saw many historical places and things I had read about during my Chinese schooling days. I have since been to different parts of China about 10 times.

My promotion to a Consultant was confirmed in 1978. Two years later, in 1980, I was persuaded at the last minute by the "young Turks" in the hospital as well as in private practice to agree to nomination and be elected the inaugural President of the Singapore Psychiatric Association (SPA). The SPA was formed to join the establishment of the ASEAN Federation of Psychiatry and Mental Health (AFPMH) in 1981, initiated by Prof. Kusumanto Setyonegoro of Indonesia. (He can be considered the father of Asean psychiatry.) So, I became a founding council member of AFPMH as well. The member countries then were Indonesia, Malaysia, the Philippines, Thailand and Singapore. I stood down after one year to pass on the baton to my young, energetic and capable colleague, Dr. Tan Chue Tin. When the Master of Medicine in Psychiatry (MMed Psychiatry) course started in the early 1980s, I was involved in teaching, training and examining the candidates. Then, the University appointed me as a Clinical Associate Professor. The title "Prof" has stuck till today. I have certainly come a long way in my time.

I took upon myself the responsibility of initiating new medical officers posted in to do psychiatry. However, I got tired of briefing batches of new doctors over and over again on procedures, assessments and the management of psychiatric patients. I decided to write a manual for them and save myself from tiresome repetition. My first manual was typed on 12 pages of A4-sized paper and stapled at one corner. At that time, there was only one personal secretary who served the Medical Superintendent (MS). Dr. Teo Seng Hock, the MS, and the Hospital Secretary, together wore many hats and performed the roles and duties of CEO, COO, CFO, HR and PRO. In addition, the MS was also the CMB (Chairman of Medical Board), a Clinical Unit Head, chief examiner of postgraduate psychiatry, and a fully active clinician providing consultations, seeing new patients, and following up on outpatients. He even made night spot checks in the hospital. His loyal personal secretary, Agnes Suriya, was kind enough to assist us in typing our articles and reports as we did not have a personal secretary. Others had to go to the typists in the common pool. Agnes had started with a manual typewriter and got quite excited when electric typewriters became available. For duplicating/printing, texts were typed on wax paper, which was then placed over a roller with ink, and copies were made on blank paper. The process was known as "cyclostyling". It could get very messy and dirty when the black ink spilled or leaked. Errors typed on the wax paper could be erased by covering mistakes with red ink or wax and typed over when dry. It was laborious. We also used transparency sheets for teaching.

Then the computer came. I revised my text about every two years and learned to type on my own, using at first Word Star, then Lotus Notes and WordPerfect, and finally, Microsoft Word. Our colleagues, Drs. Chew Sek Kee and Leong Oil Ken, were our gurus in computer and troubleshooting. The notes eventually became *Guide to Psychiatry* in thin booklets, which later grew thicker over the years into a small guidebook. It gets updated every two to three years, with the 15th revision coming out in 2017. Lundbeck generously printed hundreds of copies for distribution without obligation. In the 1990s, I also co-authored with Prof. Kok Lee Peng from NUS, Department of Psychological Medicine, and Prof. Molly Cheang from the Law Faculty, two forensic books: *Diminished Responsibility: With Special Reference to Singapore* and *Mental Disorders and the Law*.

In 1983, I was involved in the sensational Adrian Lim case of ritual murders. Lim and his two female accomplices had killed two young children under the guise of Hinduism and occult art practice. As one victim was a Malay boy, the case became a sensitive racial and religious issue. Three sets of senior lawyers and consultant psychiatrists represented the three accused because the issue of mental disorder was raised. Mental disorder was frequently invoked as a defense for diminished responsibility to escape the death sentence. I was the sole expert witness for the prosecution, working together with Glen Knight, the sole Deputy Public Prosecutor. The court hearing went on for weeks with daily reports in all the newspapers. It was very stressful and tiring to be cross-examined for days on the stand. During the trial, I overheard one day that the top people in the government were concerned and asked the Medical Superintendent how I was coping. He reassured me that I was doing all right. In the end, I was quoted verbatim in my opinion of Lim by the presiding Judge Sinnathuray that "He (Adrian Lim) has been purposeful in his pursuits, patient in his planning and persuasive in his performance for personal power and pleasure". The three accused were convicted. I did not feel inflated. In a murder trial where a conviction could lead to hanging, there was no such thing as "winning or losing the case", for a medical witness's vocation is to cure, care and comfort. After the trial, three different books by different authors were written on the Adrian Lim case.

Soon after the trial, I went on a fellowship under the Ministry of Health refresher scheme to the USA, Japan and Hong Kong in 1984. It was equivalent to the present-day HMDP (Health Manpower Development Plan). I spent one month in each place. In the USA, I spent three weeks in New York and one week in Los Angeles (LA). I put up with Dr. Stephanie Chew, a former doctor in Woodbridge Hospital in New Jersey, and Mr. Wong Kum Seng in LA. I visited their hospitals, institutes of research (Nathan Kline) and centres, e.g., Rockland of Mental Health. They had begun using computers for hospital and clinical operations 20 years ahead of us. There were all sorts of mental health programmes and facilities. Groups for all kinds of problems and conditions were formed for treatment and support. Management models were largely developed and practiced in universities and research centres, but not quite across the board for everyone. They had impressive lists of staff where almost everybody was a professor. I later learned from my daughter that assistant professors were probably lecturers and associate professors were probably senior lecturers in the British system. Through my contacts, newspaper readings and TV watching, I observed that everybody in the USA advertised and promoted themselves and competed with one another. It was puzzling that, as a supposedly Christian country, where Christianity teaches humility, modesty, service, and not to let one hand know of the other hand in charity, this self-aggrandisement was prevalent. To be fair, it applied to both positive and negative matters.

In Japan, I spent three weeks in Tokyo and one week in Sapporo. I stayed in the Singapore Embassy in Roppongi through a recommendation from Dr. Lim Hsin Loh, a son-in-law of Wee Kim Wee, who had been an ex-ambassador in Japan and later President of Singapore. I visited their hospitals and universities. The neuropsychiatrists, as they called themselves, were active in research. They had their own laboratories and used electronic microscopes and handled chromatographs expertly. They would source the brains of animals and then freeze, slice and stain the tissues themselves. They were innovative in psychogeriatric management and had volunteers from housewives. Space was at a premium in the hospital, and doctors did their work from small tables along the corridors. The office cum common room was small and shared with one another. It was crowded and stuffy because they also smoked heavily. During a case presentation, the patient's case history was written on white paper on a board. Although I did not know Japanese, I was able to follow because half or more of the words were in Chinese, though grammatically different. There were no formal courses and examinations for psychiatry. A doctor could just spend two years of attachment in a psychiatric department and qualify to practice as a psychiatrist. A small number, academically inclined, would do the 5-year research work with a dissertation for a doctorate in science (DSc). An interesting observation was that the more a doctor prescribed, the more money he would get paid. As a result, polypharmacy was common. During the last week, I flew up north to Sapporo. It was cold and snowing. Clark University, where I was to stay, sent a senior psychiatrist to meet me at the airport. He had with him three overcoats, sized small, medium and large, waiting for me. I was simply overwhelmed by the thoughtfulness and hospitality. At the end of my Japanese course, my family came over to join me for a holiday tour of Japan.

My last leg was in Hong Kong, my second home by now. My family and I stayed with my in-laws. Hong Kong, being a British colony, shared many similarities with Singapore in psychiatry. However, they were advanced in community psychiatry and rehabilitation. Part of the reason I suspected was due to their crammed housing situation. The Hong Kong Jockey Club played a very important part. They had a lot of funds and provided strong financial support to outpatient psychiatric services. The Jockey Club was like our Totalisator Board. Overall, I have gained much insight.

In 1996, I received the Public Administration Medal (Silver) on National Day Awards. The citation for the award was as follows:

> *Dr. Chee Kuan Tsee, a man with a great passion for psychiatry, has had more than 30 years' association with IMH/WH. He was appointed Head of Unit III in the seventies, and the Head of General Psychiatry in 1993 when the hospital moved to its present site and underwent a*

re-organisation of the clinical departments. He was formerly a Clinical Associate Professor with the National University of Singapore (NUS).

For the past 3 decades, he has been a respected and much sought after teacher of medical students, psychiatrists, nurses, and allied health professionals like psychologists, occupational therapists and medical social workers. His deliberations on the philosophy of life and psychiatry are profound and thought provoking. In this respect, he is often invited as the plenary speaker for both local and regional psychiatric conferences. Since the establishment of the Master of Medicine in Psychiatry in 1983, he has been both a teacher of Basic Specialist Trainees and Advanced Specialist Trainees, and an Internal Examiner for the Master of Medicine in psychiatry examination.

Apart from his collection of research papers written over the years, Dr. Chee has co-authored two well-known books on Forensic Psychiatry, which are used as reference in local context: 'Diminished Responsibility (with special reference to Singapore)' and 'Mental Disorders and The Law'. He also wrote a book entitled 'Guide to Psychiatry for Medical Officers (WH)' and he updates it regularly for the benefit of the junior doctors.

In the field of professional development, he blazed the trail to be the Inaugural President of the Singapore Psychiatric Association in 1980. He also served as an Inaugural Council Member of the Federation for Psychiatry and Mental Health (ASEAN) in 1981, and past Chairman of the Chapter of Psychiatrists, Academy of Medicine, Singapore. A fatherly figure, Dr. Chee has shaped many generations of psychiatrists in Singapore. He has dedicated his entire career to IMH/WH and truly embodies our values.

Dr. Chee is best known for his passion for teaching and imparting his knowledge and skills to generations of psychiatrists who have benefited from his vast experience.

Colleagues and patients alike have discerned, beyond his forthright manner, his genuine care and concern for them and know that he always has their best interest at heart. He is widely regarded as a person of integrity who speaks his mind and practices what he preaches.

Although he retired in 1997, he continued to work full time to help mentor the young doctors. Such was his dedication to the profession that despite suffering a heart attack in 2003 and undergoing revascularisation surgery, he continued to work on a part-time basis from September 2003.

He stayed with staff during the quarantine period in May 2003 and even volunteered to do night duty calls as we were short of doctors. He was the first doctor in IMH to be conferred the title of 'Emeritus Consultant' in 2003 in light of his distinguished service and contribution to the hospital.

When he received his salary adjustment in Jan 2003, he decided to donate the entire quantum of adjustment to WH Endowment Fund monthly. When IMH opened our Juiceworks (a mini health bar which was managed by our patients) outlet in July 2004, he was one of the first in the line who purchased food items from them. We can always count on his support towards the cause for our patients. He is generous but remains humble despite all.

Dr. Chee is also well regarded for his compassion. He had, in the past, participated in an overseas medical mission to help a third-world country. He looks out for his subsidised patients by assisting them in whatever way he can, and he is known to support his fellow psychiatrists when necessary.

Psychiatry can be considered a relatively 'young' medical specialty in Singapore with only 100 psychiatrists strewn in the public and private sectors. Dr. Chee who is one of the pioneers of psychiatry in Singapore, is looked up to as a respected teacher, sound doctor, solid family man, as well as a citizen with a heart.

I officially retired from service in 1997 when I turned 60 years old. But I continued to be on full-time re-employment and was conferred the title of Emeritus Consultant in early 2003/2004. Credit goes to Dr. Luisa Lee, the new CEO of IMH/WH, for her nomination. Soon after, the terrible SARS (severe acute respiratory syndrome) epidemic came to Singapore. There was initial panic, but we quickly organised procedures and protocols to contain its spread. There were close monitoring of fever and infection and the movement of persons. People were quarantined when necessary. Everybody and all aspects of life in Singapore were affected. The whole country was galvanised into action and precautions. At WH/IMH, I was on roster to man the Emergency Department to keep admissions to a minimum to reduce the risk of infection coming in from the outside. We could not go home. I had not done night duties for years, and it was a struggle. But the most stressful thing for me was to gown up with protective clothes, headgear, mask, gloves and boots. I could hardly breathe. We were fortunate to be spared SARS in WH/IMH. Notwithstanding, 238 persons had been infected, and 33 died, including a few doctors in Singapore.

In 2008, I received the Lee Foundation-National Healthcare Group Lifetime Achievement Award. The honour was a great surprise to me. I was grateful to the CEO then, Mr. Leong Yew Meng, for the nomination.

In 2016/2017, the College of Psychiatrists, Academy of Medicine, Singapore, was established. The predecessor was the Chapter of Psychiatrists, and I was the second Chairman in 1987/1988. The founding President of the College of Psychiatrists was Dr. Ng Beng Yeong, who was the author of *Till the Break of Day*, a history of Mental Health Services in Singapore 1841–1993. Together with Dr. Daniel Fung, they wrote *Mental Health of a Nation*, published in 2018, to update the history. He called me in early 2017 to tell me about the College's decision on the Inaugural Chee Kuan Tsee Lecture and whether I would accept. I felt honoured and humbled. In May 2017, the lecture was delivered by Dr. Benjamin Ong, Director of Medical Services, Ministry of Health, in the presence of some

40 members and colleagues. The Second Lecture was delivered in March 2019, and then subsequently annually.

In October 2017, I completed 50 years of service in IMH/WH, albeit the last 14 years were part-time, i.e., 21 hours a week after my heart attack in 2003.

Medical History and Related Services

When SARS was over, I quickly booked my leave to go to New Zealand for a break, but before I left, I had a severe attack of pain in my abdomen, which I failed to recognise as angina. I once had similar but milder transient abdominal pains dating back to the Adrian Lim case in 1983. I would describe those pains as an expanding and stretching sensation in the stomach rather than constricting pain in the chest. Also, I did not want to disappoint Kiter, who had been worried and stressed when we were dealing with SARS. We flew to Christchurch for our holiday in May 2003, when the weather was still mildly cold. We arranged for a trip to go down south. I was all right the first few days. One morning, while walking on a glacier, the pain came back and persisted. I could not go on walking but did not realise that I had a heart problem. My wife went to look for help as I was pale and sweating. A nurse from Canada, who happened to be also a tourist, told me, "I think you are having a heart attack." She quickly went around to the other tourists and found two tablets of aspirin for me. My wife found a couple of Britons to keep watch on me while she went to look for the guide, who called for a sightseeing helicopter in the area to come. Two men carried me physically into the "bubble" helicopter and flew me and Kiter to a nearby rural clinic, which operated only once a week and happened to be open on that very day. The general practitioner on duty took my history, did an ECG, and confirmed that I had an acute myocardial infarct. He gave me a morphine injection and oxygen and arranged for an ambulance helicopter to fly me to the nearest general hospital in Greymouth. I was put on a stretcher in the helicopter. There was no place for my wife, but a police patrol car happened to be around, and the police officer offered to fetch her to Greymouth because he was on his way there. Meanwhile, the guide had gone to the hotel to collect our luggage and make arrangements for checking out.

Once in Greymouth, I was handed over to the waiting medical staff. The pilot (or crew member) passed me a piece of paper to sign and departed without mentioning anything. Routine history and physical examination were carried out, and my blood was taken for tests. I was admitted straightaway to the intensive care ward. There were three beds in the small ward, separated by curtains. Another patient, one bed away, was rather talkative and noisy. Dr. Green, who happened to be a visiting cardiologist from Auckland, attended to me. He was friendly, kind and reassuring. Throughout this period, I was somehow calm and detached. I was just like a naive layman, but my wife was understandably worried and stressed. The police officer brought her to the hospital, and she checked into a motel across the road. I was in the intensive care ward for three days. The nursing staff was most caring and comforting. I also learned that the kiwi fruit was very good for constipation. They dispensed it as chilled kiwi fruit squash. The policeman who drove my wife to the hospital met her in the supermarket the day after my admission. He enquired about my health. A priest who saw my name on the hospital patient list also offered his consolations and prayers. On the 4th day, I was moved to the common ward. About three days later, I was discharged from the hospital and moved over to the motel across the road. I still needed to go back to the hospital for the monitoring and titration of warfarin, a blood anticoagulant. Our daughter, Yung En, took leave and flew over from Melbourne to be with us.

On discharge, Dr. Green spoke to me. He told me that I had a moderately severe heart attack and that my cardiac function was half that of a normal heart (but I could still eat a good cut of steak once a fortnight). He also encouraged me to get a car and drive around to see a bit of New Zealand! Such was his concern for my quality of life. Indeed, we did rent a car, and Yung En drove us to little towns and scenic spots nearby, as well as Hokitika, a rather arty town. She was also a good cook of delicious dishes. One evening, Kiter and I went for my walking exercise in the neighbourhood. I stopped intermittently to rest. A little boy of 7 or 8 years old came up to ask whether we were lost and offered help. We were touched and assured him that we were alright. Earlier, a nurse had offered to drive my wife to the supermarket.

Before we left Greymouth, we went back to the hospital to thank the staff and say goodbye. We asked for the hospital bill. The staff in charge told us to go home first and not to worry! We left our address. We took the train back to Christchurch through the "Scenic Alps" of New Zealand. We stayed in a hotel in Christchurch for a few days while Kiter made arrangements with SIA to upgrade me to business class. Meanwhile, I went out to the city, walked in the snow and even ate ice cream. We met a former colleague, Dr. Dominic Lim, and his parents, who showered care and hospitality on us. Our daughter returned to Melbourne after making sure that we could manage on our own. Despite the heart attack, it was the most memorable experience of the hospitality and kindness of people in New Zealand.

Back in Singapore, I quickly made an appointment to see the cardiologist, Prof. Chia Boon Lock, a friend. When he heard my account of what happened, he exclaimed that it was like a Hollywood drama and that I was lucky to have survived. An angiogram was quickly arranged and carried out by a younger cardiologist, Dr. Tan Huay Cheem. It was an unhappy experience and memory. Before I reached the theatre, I was asked about payment and reminded of the charges by staff at three stations, even though I repeatedly informed them that I was a pensioner holding the Singapore Civil Service Card. Then, on the operating table in the cold theatre, I was partially naked and casually covered with a blanket and was shivering. Perhaps the catheterisation was carried out through the femoral route in the groin, so my private parts were fully exposed. I had a minor angina attack during the process. I was told that I had only three coronary arteries, and two were blocked. The senior cardiologist, Prof. Chia, helped me to decide on the spot to go for stents rather than a bypass. Later, he even commented that if the 3rd artery had also been blocked, then that was it. He also mentioned that I had been given the gold standard of medication in New Zealand. I was quite ill after the procedure and had to be observed and monitored in the intensive care ward. A senior registrar came in the middle of the night to make a check. He was cold and perfunctory and did not say a word. Yet, I was a senior colleague.

Although I had enjoyed myself in Christchurch before I flew back, I felt weak and tired after the treatment. The CEO, Leong Yew Meng, surmised that my heart attack was brought on by the stress during SARS. He told me that I could be on medical leave for as long as I needed and not to worry. He was an alumnus of Chinese High School and considered me to be his senior, even at work. I received many phone calls and get-well cards, even when I was in New Zealand. Friends and colleagues visited me at home. When I finally resumed duty after a few weeks, I decided to go part-time and stop seeing new referrals — I had enough old and regular patients on follow-up to keep me occupied. I have kept myself active by reflecting, thinking, writing, teaching, providing consultation, as well as learning. I shall include and share some of my thoughts and writings in the second section that I have published in my *Guide to Psychiatry*, 15th Revision, which has been for internal circulation, so far.

Now, I should go back to my medical bills in New Zealand. I needed to make insurance claims. But there was no news from Greymouth. I wrote to them, and they replied that they had no system of charging. I explained to them my situation with the insurance, and they replied that, in that case, they would charge a hotel rate for my hospitalisation. A few weeks later, the helicopter service sent me their bill. I paid up promptly. The company thanked me for paying up and even sent me by airmail a videotape of the glacier tour to make up for what we had missed. Together with the quality of life that Dr. Green had emphasised and encouraged, it was quite a contrast with my experience back home.

In 2004, I was hospitalised in NUH for five days with lobar pneumonia of influenza A. I had a high fever for three days but had no chest pain or breathlessness. I was told that I could have died. It was probably true in view of my age and heart condition. The year after, I was seized with severe pain in my back when I woke up one morning. I could hardly bend over the sink or put on my pants. The orthopaedic surgeon diagnosed me with lumbar spondylosis after the MRI. I was given analgesics or painkillers and referred to the physiotherapist. I was also told that it would flare up now and then, which it has. I have helped myself so far with stretching exercises taught to me by a general practitioner and swimming 20 laps or 1 km continuously twice a week, then

10 laps, and now 6 laps. However, the pain and stiffness are still there every morning upon waking up or from lying down, but they fade away during the activities of the day.

Concluding Miracles and Celebrations

One of the last, but not least, miracles concerns my father's conversion to Christianity. My father was a Confucianist with a strong sense of family kinship and tradition. Our old house was like a Chee Clan family house, as mentioned earlier. His brothers and families would stay with us on and off for short periods of time. When he became the surviving patriarch of the Chee Clan, 50–60 family members and relatives would come to pay respects every Chinese New Year and exchange greetings and "ang pows" (gift of money in red packets). During Chinese New Year eves as well as my parents' birthdays, his children and their families would bring a variety of cooked food for a grand potluck dinner.

My father aside, our family was Christian by faith. It started with my maternal grandmother, who first converted. My mother had gotten us all baptised when we were children, and in the Anglican Church tradition, we had to make our own commitment and promise when we were 12 years or older for confirmation by the Bishop. My father was anti-Christian rather than against Christianity. He opined that Christian behaviour fell short of Biblical teachings. So, we were cautious about preaching to him. However, he did not interfere with our faith and church activities. As a matter of fact, he enjoyed the family celebration every Christmas Eve and ate heartily, listening to the traditional carols being sung. He had not done any work after he retired at 55 years old, but he kept up with current affairs, reading the newspaper and watching TV daily, and gave his comments. We celebrated our parents' 71st wedding anniversary at the Fullerton Hotel with an overnight stay for them. My nephew, Xufan, an operatic baritone, and his sister, Xuan, a choir soprano, flew back from the USA to sing for them at the dinner reception. Their mother, Amy, played on the electric organ. We chose the Fullerton Hotel because it had housed the colonial government offices in the past, as well as the General Post Office. My father had worked and retired there. Soon after, my father suffered from strokes, a chest infection, and a weak heart. He had hardly ever sought medical treatment in the past and always believed in natural healing and deep breathing. But during the last two years of his life, he had been in and out of hospital. We called the priest, Revd. Freddy Tan, to talk to him and pray for him. He did not object. About three weeks before he passed away at 98 years old, he asked to be baptised. We were overjoyed for his salvation and thanked God for His great love, grace and mercy. Our priest, Revd. Lim Kek Hwa, preached of the labourers of the vineyard who were employed late in the day but received the same wage as those who started work in the early morning from the owner, at his funeral. It was a most appropriate sermon. Less than two years later, my mother passed away at the age of 94. She had lived a full life. She had been a very stoic person and loved travelling. Despite her multiple medical conditions, she had been to the UK thrice to visit her younger brother, Kim, and to attend my sister's and a nephew's graduation, respectively. She had also been to the USA a few times to visit my youngest brother, David, who was then working in the church there. I had also taken her in a wheelchair to Beijing.

In the early part of 2014, I attended my first medical class reunion after 48 years. I never felt I belonged to the class and, therefore, class reunions did not mean much to me, but this time, with the persuasion of a few classmates and Kiter, I decided to put aside my own hang-ups of the past and went to Cha Am/Hua Hin, Thailand. It turned out to be enjoyable and memorable. Many classmates came from Malaysia and Singapore, but there were also those who had migrated to Australia and the USA. Although I have not seen many for years, we still remembered one another.

In November 2016, the medical class of 1966 celebrated our Golden Jubilee in Singapore, where it all began for us. There were nearly 90 of us, including spouses. Many were not in good health, and one passed away a few weeks later. I missed the reunion in September 2017 in Cameron Highlands because of my back pain, which had flared up. However, in November 2017, I recovered well enough, and the whole family went together to Melbourne and Tasmania for our long-overdue family bonding holiday. We had a great time seeing the mountains, valleys, and the coasts. We enjoyed Cradle Mountain in Tasmania and, in particular, the spread of food. Now, there is a plan for my classmates to meet again in Perth in the future.

As a matter of fact, to celebrate our 40 years of marriage, Kiter and I went to Western Australia in 2014. Yung En flew over from Melbourne and drove us and her friend to many national parks to see the scenery and particularly the wildflowers everywhere, which Kiter loved. We also went to Hong Kong for a reunion with relatives. At the same time, Kiter attended the 50th anniversary of St. Rose Convent, her secondary school celebration. In January 2018, she attended the 70th anniversary of her school. Incidentally, she was the founding president of the alumni.

Since the passing of our parents, my brothers, sister and I have been meeting weekly for lunch, and our families also celebrate Christmas and Chinese New Year together at the family house where my younger sister lives.

God has blessed us all abundantly and has planned and guided our lives throughout the years. The miracles in my life are evidence. In some ways, the miracles in my life mirror the miracles of Singapore in its independence, growth and development of the last 50 years and more.

I tell people that I owe all my achievements in life to my mother before I got married and my wife, Kiter, after our marriage. Of course, above all, God has made all things possible and blessed us all with the miracles in life.

I hope that I shall be able to continue to count the blessings and give thanks.

I started writing my story in SG50 when ex-Deputy Prime Minister Heng Swee Kiat encouraged people to write their stories, but I stopped halfway. Now that it is SG60, I decided to pick it up again after I fully retired in 2025. There may be some updating here and there.

Publication of my Books

My book *Guide to Psychiatry: Singapore Perspective*, 16th Revision, was published in 2020/2021 by World Scientific Publishing. The earlier revisions were printed by pharmaceutical firms for free distribution to medical staff and allied healthcare colleagues. The decision to publish was for a wider readership. All royalties are to go to Woodbridge Hospital Charity Fund, which is the sole beneficiary. The book so far has received favourable reviews.

As mentioned in the earlier citation on "Emeritus Consultant", I have co-authored two forensic books, *Diminished Responsibility: With Special Reference to Singapore* and *Mental Disorders and the Law*, with Prof. Kok Lee Peng, a psychiatrist, and Prof. Molly Cheang in Law.

Section II

Reflections on Governance and Management in the Course of Working Experience

Most of my thoughts in this section come from the last three chapters of my book *Guide to Psychiatry: Singapore Perspective*, 16th Revision, published in 2020 by World Scientific Publishing.

The Nature of Psychiatry

The Brain and the mind are inseparable. The human person has physical, psychological, social and spiritual attributes, which are **interrelated, interactive and integrated in structure and function**. Mental disorder is **multifactorial in causality** and **multidisciplinary in management**. The **biopsychosocial model** is more **holistic** and **integrative** than **eclectic** and **combining** in nature and approach. It is the **developmental** and **dynamic inter-relation, interaction and integration versus pathological dissociation** between:

1. Individual and environmental — genes, relationships, work, crises, stress and disasters
2. Body/brain and mind — physical and psychological systems
3. Neuro-circuitries and mental functions — neurotransmitters, synapses and wiring

4. Past and present events and experiences — memory trauma and influence
5. Chain reactions — in continuous stimulus-response
6. In addition, it depends on and what is "**downloaded**" in education, social media, policy and concepts of democracy, human rights, freedom of speech, globalisation, lifestyle, digital technology and artificial intelligence (AI), etc. In many ways, the functions or faults in a computer reflect the workings of the brain and mind in both the conscious and unconscious realms.

In the course of my work and career at Woodbridge Hospital (WH) (1967–1993) and the Institute of Mental Health (IMH) (1993–2025), I have encountered the fallout (or causality) from changes and crises in people's lives and our society. Extended families living in kampongs were broken up when they were moved into high-rise HDB flats. Older folks were especially affected and stressed in their new environments. Hainanese women, who spoke only Hainanese, felt isolated and depressed. Dialect-speaking churches and clan associations dwindled in their memberships. In the process of nationalising our education system, Chinese-speaking teachers were handicapped. They had to switch to teaching in English and had to learn how to use the computer. Many were stressed and could not cope. They became burned out, anxious and depressed, and we had to medical-board several of them out from the teaching service so that they would not lose their pension and medical benefits. Some returned to teach free from stress as they had the choice and control to stop anytime without loss when they could not cope. It was not a case of malingering as some had deemed. During the Lehman Brothers financial crisis, some patients remarked that what they needed was a blank cheque and not expensive antidepressant drugs. What did help, I believe, was when the banks were told to do the right thing about investor losses. Our patients, who were used to single-storey wards with ample open grounds to freely roam and play about, had difficulty adjusting when they were moved into the multi-storey locked-up wards of the new WH/IMH in 1993. In psychiatry, linguistic proficiency and skill are most important in communication and taking good history between the doctor, patient and management. But many of our younger generations of medical staff, as well as foreign recruits, could only speak English and Mandarin. I had to assist in translation because I could speak Hokkien, Teochew, Cantonese, and my mother tongue, Foochow, and had some working command of Malay. Because of this language barrier, the older generation was also unable to pass down cultural customs and values.

In a way, through our contacts with patients and people, we can say that we have our finger on the **pulse of the nation**. For instance, many of our HDB dwellers survive on the rentals of their rooms or flats, although foreign workers are required to pay heavily. The not-so-educated end up working as cleaners with low wages, and the better-educated work as security guards with long hours or as private hire drivers. Many also live and enjoy in advance on credit or by depending on their parents.

Upon reflection, I would like to share my observation and experience on the importance of **"active balance and passive equilibrium"** in life.

It seems there are **four major areas** of **conflict, tension** and **stress** in modern living. They are not mutually exclusive and, in fact, overlap and interplay. What is discussed below is with special reference to psychotherapy. Indeed, these conflicts or dilemmas are applicable to other things.

A. Evolutionary Processes versus Revolutionary Changes

Biological development is evolutionary in nature, and its functioning is integrative. There is a built-in feedback mechanism that monitors the organism's internal and external environments continuously. The processes generally follow a predictable course and time span. Thus, the growth and development of a child go through defined stages. Education and training take time, and specialisation takes even more time. There is no way to mass produce precious personnel in a shorter time by way of mechanisation, computerisation and automation, the key processes in productivity. Hence, the import of foreign talents when needs arise. However, intended expertise is not transferred and maximised and reliance on foreign talents is perpetuated. The biased practice or inbreeding of work culture takes place and becomes a problem. Meanwhile, the local workforce may or may not be ready in upskilling and is picky, impatient and feels displaced and resentful.

Social changes, on the other hand, are man-made and tend to be ad hoc and lopsided, addressing specific problems and needs or wants during certain periods of time. In our competitive world, they occur so rapidly that our biological makeup cannot match the pace. A concrete example would be the phenomenon of jet lag when our physiological rhythm is out of step with a change in time zone. The necessity for shift duties, especially the third shift, apart from social implications, can also upset the body systems with regard to sleep, appetite and bowel habits. It is not surprising that sleeping pills and alcohol are used to overcome the problem of insomnia. Frequent or constant abrupt changes of policy and organisation disrupt people in their long-term plans and commitments. This is made worse by incredible advances in digital technology disruption. Old jobs are destroyed, and new jobs are created. Soon, foreign talents or workers will be replaced by computers, machines and robots.

Biological adaptation takes time, and the learning process is arduous — it cannot be reversed or switched on and off at will. The ageing older generation or elderly persons suffer because they have greater difficulty coping with rapid changes, acquiring new know-how, or undergoing re-training. Even the conversion to the metric system, e.g., in North America, has been a laborious or deliberate process and has taken years to complete or is yet to be fully converted. Cultural attitudes, beliefs and customs are not changed overnight by economic success or scientific discovery. The human mind may reach into the sky to be among the gods, but the human heart is still in the jungle with the animals.

Implications for psychotherapy

Modern living is fast-paced and changing, characterised by the instant culture of constant stimulation, seduction and self-indulged gratification of fad and fashion, the Internet, sex, drugs, computer games, virtual or metaverse reality, AI, etc. However, psychotherapy takes time, and the individual needs time, but changes do not keep time. Personality traits are also enduring.

On the other hand, deep-rooted cultural beliefs and practices are not to be underestimated for their therapeutic roles — they can be an ally or an enemy in therapy.

B. Role Prescription/Acceptance versus Individual Right/Freedom

In the Confucian society, there is an **ethical code of conduct** and a **hierarchy of social organisation** that must be strictly observed. Everybody knows his station in life and lives according to his **multiple roles and relationships**, i.e., as a ruler, citizen, employer, employee, friend, father, son, brother, husband, etc. He acts and responds dutifully in line with expectation, and there is rule and order. Naturally, this is subject to a complete and willing acceptance of prescribed roles and relationships inculcated from young. The elders must always be respected, and their words are law. Young men and women who have come of age must marry, and the go-between is asked to look for compatible matches. The greatest sin of unfilial piety is not to produce a male heir to carry on the family name. For the female, she must follow her father before she is married, follow her husband when she is married, and follow her son when she is widowed. She must also be virtuous in her conduct, appearance, speech and work. There seems to be no place for self-identity and expression. It is to be expected that there will be sufferings and tragedies, mostly because of **human weakness** and **wickedness** rather than the system itself, **for roles and relationships are abused and exploited for selfish ends by those in positions of power.**

In Christian teaching, the wife is to obey the husband, but the husband is also to love his wife. In marriage, the two become one and are not separated by the inequality of gender.

With exposure to Western philosophy and its way of life, men and women apparently liberate themselves from social restrictions and claim their **rights as individuals** to seek self-fulfilment or do as they please. The gender of a person or his/her "seniority" does not seem to matter much. In Western society, people call one another by personal name regardless of differences in hierarchy and generation. This reduces all relationships to a linear one of apparent equality and contributes to social chaos. Conflict arises when his/her **expression of freedom** is at odds with his/her **social obligations**. It becomes disastrous when he/she cannot handle his/her freedom responsibly and abuses it like a cancer in society. Inevitably, respect for law and order and traditional wisdom breaks down. Schism and alienation set in. Seniority and experience count for nothing. The filial children of yesterday become unwanted parents of today. The new idolatry is indiscriminate **individualism**.

Of course, man would like to believe that he is enlightened through education and religion. However, cruelty, corruption and crime still abound everywhere. Only the form and method have become more sophisticated. Countries are divided among themselves by ideology, race, language and religion. They kill each other in the loftiest proclamation. The violence of exploding bombs, the greed in drug trafficking, and the exploitation of sex, regardless of consequences and conscience, should complete the scenario. Human nature over the ages has been unchanging. Ironically, the result of democracy is dictators or oligarchy. However, to shackle a person into rigid roles is as dangerous and tragic as to give free rein to his passions.

Implications for psychotherapy

Whether we admit it or not, we play **multiple roles** and interact at **many levels** all the time, consciously or unconsciously. At different times, there may be a dominant role and other subsidiary roles in different situations; for example, the doctor and patient roles in a clinical setting are dominant roles. When other roles creep in between them, transference is said to have taken place, and the relationship is changed. The **upbringing of children is**

in conflict and confusion of values and virtues in different cultures, societies, research evidence and theories.

It is often forgotten that the **relationship** between two persons changes with a change in roles, e.g., as lovers, as husband and wife and as parents. Furthermore, the characteristics or expectations of each role also undergo changes, e.g., a stereotyped gender role. Each society has its own concept of the necessity and expectation of roles.

However, certain hierarchical roles are unalterable in real life. People do not just relate and interact as equal individuals but also observe their social stations of wealth and poverty. There is a genuine **conflict** between preserving family structure and functioning and establishing individual identity and independence. **Stephen Fleck** said many years ago that "**when roles and relationships are well defined and fulfilled, stability and satisfaction in the family life can be expected**".

C. Consumerism versus Conservationism

There is a cliché that change in life is constant, but the reality is that human nature, of selfishness, greed, corruption and cruelty, is unchanging. In the race to create wealth, the environment is exploited, the world is polluted by excess waste, and the climate is changing, which endangers all species, including human beings. To control and curb the complex and ingenious human commissions and omissions, there have been proliferations of rules and regulations, protocols and procedures, and laws and ethics, which are not universally observed. Digital technology and AI are churned out continuously to create more "wants" than "needs" to flood the markets to satisfy insatiable gratification. The new products and services are incessantly promoted and propagated by businesses and the mass media, quickly become outdated and obsolete and then discarded. Stress in life continues in competition.

It is useful to remember the mnemonic of the idol **MAMMONISM:**

Make money by hook or by crook
Accumulate wealth beyond needs
Market consumerism as the global icon
Merge and restructure to compete and control
Optimise mastery, monopoly, and mass production
Negotiate with turn and twist and to give little away
Interfere and destabilise, then exploit for gains
Sins are to be whitewashed for survival or success
Money is the alpha and omega (or the secular "God")

Implications for psychotherapy

We need to resolve the intra-psychic conflicts of individual development and growth, and the external conflicts of human survival needs of the world at large. Human behaviour is determined by biological instincts, social influences, and legal controls or unilateral hegemony. They must be reconciled in balance.

D. Survival of the Misfits and Unfits (and Unwilling)

It should be stated from the outset that the right to survival is unquestionable. The terms "misfits" and "unfits" are not absolute and have nothing to do with the Nazi's idea of creating a super race. They are to be viewed from the perspective of the biological concept of Darwin regarding the **survival of the fittest**. In a certain sense, we are all misfits, unfits and unwilling in some ways. Our personality development is **uneven,** and we all have our strengths and weaknesses. We may be brilliant or dull in mind, beautiful or blemished in physique, and stable or volatile in temperament. An individual could be an intellectual giant but suffer from social inadequacies, sexual deviance, or emotional immaturity. To put it crudely, some people are socially high class but morally low class or intellectually first class but spiritually no class. Depending on the period and culture he/she lives in and the value system that is upheld, he/she may enjoy public prominence or languish in anonymity. (**One man's meat may be another man's poison, but what is meat today may be poison tomorrow.**) One personality may be viewed as a hero in one situation but a crook in another.

To achieve progress, we have traded **general versatility** for **intensive specialisation**. In the process, we have become more **interdependent** for mutual services and more vulnerable when such services break down or when our individual talents fail or go out of demand. On the other hand, **market forces** are such that what is in demand could dictate exorbitant terms with impunity, e.g., sports stars and performing artists. There are also very young millionaires or even billionaires with their innovations or creations that capture the world.

With advancement in medical sciences and technology, as well as the affluence of the civilised society, the **frail** and **feeble** in **body**, **mind** and **morals** have been enabled to survive. They not only survive without being productive but also expect a better quality of life and services encouraged by the welfare state. Personality disorders, mental and behavioural disorders, the abuse of psychoactive substances, the physically and intellectually disabled or handicapped, as well as the aged sick, would fall under this category. They are not only a stress to themselves as consumers but also a stress to others as providers. Incidentally, it is ironic that while fortunes are spent in modern medicine to prolong life, fortunes are also made from the sale of arms to exterminate many thriving lives. When man plays God, he must deal with the devil. The ageing population with a declining birth rate is going to be a monstrous dilemma. Fewer and fewer people who are productive will have to support more and more people who are unproductive.

Implications for psychotherapy

Psychotherapy here would have to grapple with issues of values, judgement, morality, economics and politics.

In the developed countries, the pressure is on the welfare state, but for the others, the burden is on the family.

What are the answers?

Human solutions to problems are always at the expense of something else. Every solution creates a new problem. **A price is paid by someone, somewhere, sometime**. There is no perfect or permanent solution. Nevertheless, suffering must be alleviated.

In terms of psychodynamics and treatment, Western psychotherapy aims not only to remove symptoms but also promote the growth and development of the individual. It is patient-centred, and the interest of others is of secondary importance. This is consistent with the belief that individual rights are sacrosanct. The Eastern society, however, is family-centred, and the individual is to put group interest above his/her self. For ages, the Chinese have also coped by accepting their individual fate and destiny when faced with trials and tribulations. Life is made more bearable, and individual failure or weakness is overlooked.

It may be said that the Western society encourages the vertical development of individuals that, in turn, would lift the horizontal growth of the community. However, the Eastern philosophy of life emphasises the well-being of the whole through the selfless contribution of the individuals. (Of course, there are self-centred/selfish as well as altruistic individuals in all cultures.) There is a Chinese saying that when there is no country/nation, there is no family/home. Perhaps the answer lies in the:

ACTIVE BALANCE (win-win) of **OPPOSITE VIRTUES**
and **NOT**
PASSIVE EQUILIBRIUM (zero sum) of **DOMINATION**
and **RESIGNATION**

The human community is made up of individuals, and these individuals cannot be effective without the community. Perhaps we need to **restrain the "ID" culture**, **relax the "SUPER-EGO" culture** and **reinforce the "EGO" culture**, which would hold all things together in harmony. Psychotherapy must therefore recognise the cultural norms, values and realities from which the patient comes and to which the patient returns.

Healthcare and Medical Profession and Management

In the modern world, capitalism and consumerism pervade and prevail. Multinational corporations (MNCs) are as powerful as governments, if not more so. Despite campaigns and the promotion of human rights and democracy, the gap between the haves and have-nots widens and deepens. The practice of medicine is likewise affected. In more than five decades of my medical career, I have noticed major changes in healthcare and economics and issues of policy and manpower. Worldwide, healthcare costs are escalating. Healthcare economics is very complex. Like all things, one complexity is that it has become a **commercial enterprise**. The practice of medicine has changed from one doctor treating many patients as whole persons at the primary care level to many specialists and sub-specialists managing single patients as divided body parts or even the mind at the secondary and tertiary levels. There is also a proliferation of allied health professionals or workers, technicians and managers. MNCs and private insurance schemes are profiteering and are in control.

Developing a society with limited resources would provide one-size-fits-all services that are basic. However, with development and affluence, treatment or management becomes individualised or customised. The latest investigations, machines, drugs and procedures are introduced as necessary. It becomes the new baseline of one-size-fits-all services that are expensive because of new facilities and market forces, as well as medico-legal issues and defensive practices.

People are also living longer with chronic and degenerative diseases that require long-term treatment and care. What was untreatable in the past is treatable now. There are also more diseases and disorders added because of new discoveries, changing concepts and thresholds, and the medicalisation of existential human imperfections and sufferings. In addition, there are preventive screening, early treatment and aesthetic medicine. Finally, we have so-called lifestyle diseases and disorders and addictive habits or behaviours. Mental health, wellness and illness problems are also gaining prominence and recognition.

The nature and purpose of medical education and training of future doctors have been undergoing changes and are not static. Medical practice likewise undergoes changes for better or worse. Medical schools have been revising their curricula, contents, directions and emphases, as well as tools and methods of teaching or training, e.g., problem-based learning, virtual reality. Based on the growth of knowledge and advancement in management alone, medical courses have been extended in both undergraduate (e.g., disruption for a BSc course or research project) and postgraduate studies and training, as well as lifelong continuous medical education or professional development. There is already a dilemma and tension between the balance of a broad-based generalist and the super specialist across all disciplines and subspecialists within each discipline.

The oath and pledge we take when we begin our profession are person-centred, emphasising a compassionate approach to cure, care and comfort our patients and the special fraternity within our profession. It is essential that we should constantly remind ourselves of them.

The Declaration Of Geneva (173rd WMA Council Session, Divonne-les-Bains, France May 2006 ("first" adopted by the 2nd WMA General Assembly, Geneva, Switzerland, September 1948 and amended by the 22nd WMA, Sydney, 1968; 35th WMA, Venice, October 1983; and 46th WMA General Assembly, Stockholm, September 1994; editorially revised by the 170th WMA Council Session, Divonne-les-Bains, France, May 2005) should be constantly kept in mind.

At the time of being admitted as a member of the Medical Profession:

I SOLEMNLY PLEDGE to consecrate my life to the service of humanity.

I WILL GIVE to my teachers the respect and gratitude which is their due.

I WILL PRACTISE my profession with conscience and dignity.

THE HEALTH OF MY PATIENT will be my first consideration.

I WILL RESPECT the secrets that are confided in me, even after the patient has died.

I WILL MAINTAIN by all the means in my power, the honour and the noble traditions of the medical profession.

MY COLLEAGUES will be my sisters and brothers.

I WILL NOT PERMIT considerations of age, disease or disability, creed, ethnic origin, gender, nationality, political affiliation, race, sexual orientation, social standing or any other factor to intervene between my duty and my patient.

I WILL MAINTAIN the utmost respect for human life.

I WILL NOT USE my medical knowledge to violate human rights and civil liberties, even under threat.

I MAKE THESE PROMISES solemnly, freely, and upon my honour.

However, environmental/economic factors and administrative policies have made it difficult for our oath and pledge to be fulfilled. Surprisingly, some are not fully aware of or have forgotten the substance of the oath and pledge.

We have no complete control over how we practice medicine nowadays. Administrators and management have the final say. Clinical language and terminology are replaced by business terms, such as:

Corporatisation — CEO, case manager, case-mix, customer service, cost-effectiveness, packaging and marketing, productivity, health industry and clinical technology, entrepreneurial research, medical tourism or medical hub, added value, KPI (Key Performance Index) and performance bonus and a host of other economic jargon.

Computerisation — On the one hand, facilitates management, but on the other hand, it stifles flexibility and controls how procedures should be followed. There appears to be no place for altruism. Internet-savvy consumers or clients are no longer passive patients.

There had been an error in the projection of the number and ratio of doctors needed, leading to the capping of intakes into medical schools and the restriction of recognised medical graduates from other sources. It was based on a one-size-fits-all doctor/population ratio. Demographic changes and anticipated lifestyles, e.g., ageing population, retirement, savings, family structure and support, independent living, quality of life, substance abuse, etc., probably were not taken into consideration.

We are treating what have been considered untreatable.

We are treating more and more patients with chronic conditions.

We are treating more and more conditions for marginal benefit/improvement.

We are treating more and more people because of the changing threshold criteria.

We are treating what others consider as the "medicalisation" of problems in living and habits.

We are doing things for aesthetic/cosmetic reasons and wellness promotion.

There are also preventive screening and early intervention promoted.

Also, there is attrition due to migration, retirement, sickness and death.

Finally, there is a significant influx of foreigners.

The financing of treatments through Medisave, Medishield and Medifund is continuously tweaked by policy, which is complex and confusing, although all citizens are assured of basic medical care. The controversy of different postgraduate models and programmes of training of future specialists has yet to be resolved. This has led to confusion and disparity in the assessment of proficiency and performance. There is also bound to be some unfairness to trainees in transition. On the other hand, there is also a danger of inbreeding of inherent weaknesses, inadequacies and attitudes in each scheme. The human touch, for example, is replaced by administrative correct procedures. Nevertheless, an attitude of curiosity, diligence and open-mindedness is most important. Learning from the patient is to be encouraged. In psychiatry, in particular, complacency and smugness should be guarded against strenuously. Often, it does not seem to matter whether a correct diagnosis is made or a proper treatment is given; the patient may or may not respond, is not likely to die, does not complain, and no one is wiser. To seek an answer or a solution to a problem, clinical research is necessary, besides keeping oneself updated on the latest trends, technology or treatments.

Finally, experience and skill are mostly acquired from subsidised patients in the beginning. It should benefit all and is not meant for only those who can afford it. We teach "first do no harm", that is, no harm to the body by what we do, no harm to the mind by what we say, and no harm to the pocket by what we charge. We need to ponder whether our lifestyle ought to be the by-product of what we can manage or the end-product to achieve at all costs.

Mental Health and Stress; Management and Training

Stress is part of life, but in this competitive world for survival, some people say that it is or should be a way of life for productivity and profit. Stress is, therefore, unavoidable. However, it is **not always necessary**. Very often, it is the result of incompetent, mediocre, selfish and greedy management or a personality problem. A higher or hidden reason for creating stress is perhaps to toughen up people to ensure survival, but there will be casualties, even before going to war. There are both **intrinsic** and **extrinsic factors** involved in stress. The **nature of mental health work** requires that the psychiatrist be **well-informed** and **interested** about **life.**

An MNC is occupied with the acquisition of wealth and power. Management is, therefore, focused on "making money by all means". However, this is not always fulfilled. To survive, the management resorts to "creating image" and, when necessary, attempts to "cover backside". Data is collected and analysed in the process to justify action rather than the truth. Often, any change or new introduction is not evaluated but swept under the carpet. Another set of highflyers will take over and repeat the same operation. What is more crucial than process and procedure is the quality of the people who implement.

Therefore, in our training, one should have **curiosity**, which is necessary for seeking truth and creativity; **diligence**, which is necessary for thoroughness and achievement; and an **open mind**, which is necessary for growth and development. Always ask to **clarify**, **verify**, and try to **rationalise** what we do**. To be a mentor is to be a model.**

Learn as much as possible when you are young and inexperienced.

Learn from **patients**, **know** and **understand** them and not just use them as rating scales.

Because when you become a consultant, you may be **too proud** or **shy** to learn.

And you would not be able to teach or avoid teaching what you do not know.

The worthy consultant is a **resource person** who should be humble and keep on learning.

The often-quoted **evidence-based medicine** is a **standardised** and **statistical** guide.

Its application is a bottom-line, **one-size-fits-all** approach.

Advanced or improved management would have to be **individualised** and **customised.**

This calls for **personal experience** built up **rigorously** over the years.

Evidence-based medicine is to be complemented by **experience-based medicine**, which is the original source of evidence.

Beware the power of persuasion of the pharmaceuticals, which are driven by profits.

Classification of mental disorders is **atheoretical**, **syndromal**, and, by **consensus, inclusive.**

Not all mental disorders are **diagnosable,** and they often are **forced into pigeonholes.**

Rigid adherence to the International Classification of Diseases (ICD) and, in particular, the Diagnostic and Statistical Manual of Mental Disorders (DSM), leads to **thinking in the box and stagnation.**

To seek answers or solutions to problems, **clinical research** is necessary, besides reading up. In randomised controlled trials, the larger the sample population and the longer the duration of study, the simpler the statistics will be and, more likely, the validity and reliability of the findings as well. On the other hand, the smaller the sample size and the shorter the duration of the study, the more complex the statistics will be and the less likely the validity and reliability of the results.

What Others Have Said about Science and the Art of Medicine

Treating the Bug the Patient has is Science.
Treating the Patient who has the Bug is Art.
Therefore, treating the Disease is Science and treating the Patient is Art.
To care with Competence is Science.
To care with Compassion is Art.

Best

In the best interest of the patient is not the same as giving our best.
Because our best may not be the best unless and until we become the best.

First do no harm

No harm to the body by what we do.
No harm to the mind by what we say.
No harm to the pocket by what we charge.

Cure, care, comfort

The wise physician teaches: to cure sometimes, to care often and to comfort always.
Modern medicine and technology do the reverse: to comfort sometimes, to care often and to cure always.

Change

Change in Life is said to be Constant and Continuous.

But Human Nature of Selfishness and Greed, Cruelty and Corruption is Unchanging.
Hence the proliferations of Rules and Regulations, Protocols and Procedures, Laws and Ethics.
To Control and Curb the complex and ingenious Human Commissions and Omissions.

Through my experiences at work, observations on management, understanding of human nature, and dealing with stress, I have jotted down my own **"parables"**.

The Coil Spring and the Load

Individuals are like coil springs of different materials, thickness, length and strength. Each time a weight is suspended, the spring stretches, and as the load is increased, the spring stretches proportionally. When the weight is removed, the spring returns to its original state. However, if the load keeps increasing, the spring will keep on stretching. There comes a moment when the spring does not quite return to its original position when the weight is completely taken off. This could also happen when a certain weight is applied over a prolonged or indefinite period. In this instance, the spring has undergone a qualitative change and lost its full resilience. Subsequently, its response to the force applied would be erratic and difficult to predict. Eventually, with an increasing load, a critical point is reached when the spring snaps. There is a saying about the final straw that breaks the camel's back.

Of course, an excessive weight right from the start or at any point thereafter would produce the same result in a more dramatic fashion. However, if the whole process is carried out in a different medium, i.e., immersed in a liquid, then the buoyancy effect will affect the response of the spring to the applied force.

The Horse, the Cart and the Road in Productivity

The saying about putting "the cart before the horse" refers to the wrong sequence of doing things or adopting the wrong priority. Here, we are concerned about productivity.

To carry a certain load from A to B within a certain time frame will depend on the nature of the load, the power of the horse, the size of the cart, and the conditions of the road. There are several variables in this job assignment, but we shall not discuss them all.

When the horsepower is fixed, there will be a maximum limit to the payload. The horse pulls easily when the cart is small and the load is light. More often than not, it is a full load. However, within limits, the horse can still do a good job, although its reserve may be reached. A crisis comes when the cart is overloaded or expanded to carry more, and no additional horse is available. This calls for a decision as to what valuable load should be carried and what dispensable load should be discarded. But this is not always done.

Sometimes, the horse matches the cart and the load, but the road can be narrow, winding and uneven. When a time schedule must be strictly followed, the horse and the cart head for a breakdown from exhaustion or make extra trips.

In modern IT language, we know that every computer has a fixed capacity and speed. When the diskette/hard disk is full, it cannot take in more data, but the human workforce seems to have no limit in capacity and speed to meet production targets.

The Driver and the Car

The performance of the car on the road depends not only on its roadworthiness and traffic conditions but also on the way it is driven. There are drivers who drive without changing gears or with his/her foot on the clutch or with the hand brake on. One can imagine the serious wear and tear, wastage of energy with much heat and exhaust, and the eventual breakdown of the engine and its parts. The new autopilot electric car will lead to the atrophy of a driver's skill.

"Sloggers" and "Shirkers"

With an emphasis on paper qualifications and performance measured in selective quantifiable units, the phenomenon of apparent quality and quantity emerges. Qualifications do not always predict delivery, as there are other important factors, such as personality, character, commitment, state of health, and energy level, to be considered. However, meritocracy often develops into elitism, and mistakes made at recruitment might be concealed.

Thus, on paper, the staff complement may be full. However, in reality, out of 10 persons in employment, there may be 7–8 individuals who pull their weight and 2–3 others who may not be doing their part, although all receive the same reward. To achieve maximum productivity, the 7–8 "sloggers" would have to put in extra effort to make up for the 2–3 "shirkers". A management that is concerned with increasing its output, therefore, depends more and more on the "sloggers" for their input. While the "shirkers" are allowed to get away, the "sloggers" are under stress by having to do well above their share and feeling resentful. The "sloggers" also suffer when rules are tightened with the "shirkers" in mind.

Stress is further aggravated when the management, to put it crudely, is preoccupied with "creating its image" and "covering its back", which generates unproductive activities and wastes resources. The worldly wise soon recognise that the priority is not so much to provide a better service but to please those in authority. Amazingly, feedback, monitoring, auditing and accountability appear to be satisfied merely by making rhetoric statements and submitting questionable figures. The paradoxical outcome is that the more capable an individual is, the more is expected from him/her, the more he/she is under stress, and the more likely this person will break down when he/she remains in the system, even when suitably rewarded. Stress becomes poisonous when the "slogger" works under a "shirker", whose output depends on the former's input.

Input and Output

It is not often appreciated that the output of the management depends on the input from the ground. As such, when the individual's input goes to his own output and does not directly contribute to the management's output or image, then his performance is not likely to be recognised and rewarded. Increased mechanisation, automation and computerisation are intended to increase production. But productivity depends on trained people.

In this age of IT, computerisation is an answer to efficiency and productivity. Facts and figures, when required by the management, are displayed immediately at the touch of the fingertip, but it requires enough people at the bottom to regularly collate and key in the necessary data.

Computerisation does not reduce the workforce. The user depends on the feeder. The people at the top may take minutes to formulate and issue an idea or instruction, but it takes other staff hours, days or weeks to accomplish. Often, the results are obvious, redundant or inconsequential, and much time, effort and money are wasted at the expense of other priorities. But the management must be seen to be working, and protocol must be observed.

Apart from production targets and deadlines, people can also find themselves trapped in doing things against their convictions and principles. To opt out would mean unemployment and privation.

Self-interest and Group Interest

Self-interest is innate and natural. It has survival value. The group is composed of individuals, and the group interest's should be to enhance individual interest and survival. However, there are many kinds of groups, and each group has its own purpose or function, characteristics and life. As each individual can be a member of more than one group, there will be conflicts of interest and loyalty. People have their own priorities of membership and hierarchy of group interest. Generally speaking, the one who provides work and one's livelihood is the most important.

When basic needs are satisfied, people look beyond to a higher standard of living, better working conditions, career development, job satisfaction, and being somebody. Once again, there will be conflict and tension. Stress is aggravated when group interest is divided, undermined by self-interest, or controlled by an interest outside the group. It should be noted that there could be subgroups with their own specific interests within the larger group. Sometimes, the purpose and function of the group may become outdated, and its continuity becomes a sentimental burden.

History of Corporate Stress

Corporate stress has been in existence from ancient times. There have been strong but bad rulers as well as good but weak ones. There have been ambitious and scheming courtiers who manipulated their emperors and exploited the people, and there have also been capable and virtuous statesmen who were banished or executed. In historical perspective, the enlightened dictator that is super-ego guided may be better than a dictatorship of mediocre democracy that is id driven.

In modern management and governance, the top priority is to be in control by whatever means and methods (powered perhaps by branded MBAs — Mind Brain Altered or Automated). It has been said that management creates jobs for itself and work for others. Indeed, often, the size of management grows faster than the core business manpower. The management does not contribute directly to productivity but devises ways and measurements to squeeze the workhorses to produce more. The management seems to enjoy regular travelling to get ideas, lengthy meetings to promote ideas, top-down delegating to enforce ideas, and remote controlling instead of walking the talk. What is achieved is usually "image creation" and "backside covering". It is not unlike a parasitic predator that takes control of the host and drains off much of the harvest of labour to feed its separate existence, infrastructure and running costs. (The workhorses are further squeezed to provide for the CEO's bonuses and the stakeholders' benefits.) Talent and quality or standards are dispensable if they do not meet the prevailing management culture and expectations. Therefore, for the management, it is the consolidation of power and control that really matters. For others who have acquired invaluable experience and wisdom in the course of work, they are soon discarded at a cut-off point because they are considered obstacles to the compulsive need for change and the need to make way for rejuvenation. The cycles of "3 steps forwards and 2 steps backwards" in terms of experience and wisdom are repeated as progress, as long as power and control are maintained.

Thinking in the Box

Thinking in the box is natural when it is downloaded like software on the hard disk, and one is constrained to think only of its contents. When the content is: "I know all, I know best, I decide all, I veto rest", the consequence is: "Fear to speak, Foolish to speak, Futile to speak". ISOs, SOPs and NUTS (No U-Turn Syndrome) are orders of the day. To think out of the box, we need more boxes with different contents mixing freely. However, too many short-sighted free ideas and demands may have dire long-term consequences.

Prohibition and Permissiveness

In conservative or prohibitive cultures and societies, values, attitudes, beliefs and customs are clearly spelled out. There is little ambiguity on what is good and bad, and what is right and wrong. Rules are laid down to prevent what is undesirable from taking place. People are, therefore, more inhibited. In liberal or permissive cultures and societies, the boundaries of good and bad and right and wrong are blurred. Rules are not absolute, and people are more adventurous and experimenting.

However, prohibition does not prevent what is undesirable from happening. When things do happen, the solutions to the problems are limited and restrictive. Where there is permissiveness, things are allowed to happen, and solutions are found to deal with the various problems that surface. Take, for example, the question of sex, which is associated with procreation and transmission of sexually transmitted diseases (STDs). The surest way to avoid procreation and STDs is to prohibit sex. When there is no unwanted pregnancy or STD, there is no reason to invent intervention, but when promiscuity is a way of life, one can indulge in sex without being caught, so to speak, by learning about the safe periods and the numerous methods of contraception, as well as treatments available. Open society thus seems more innovative, creative and advanced. When a closed society is faced with problems, it must look to the open society for solutions.

Innovation needs to be encouraged with support and flexibility, but it should also be tempered with conscience and caution to cause no harm.

The Economic Preoccupation

In the modern world, the new dictator that drives us on and on is materialism or consumerism. Making money has become the most important part of our culture because of its purchasing power. It can even buy talents and citizenship. There are so many things that are attractive, desirable and irresistible. Furthermore, these things are churned out so fast that they are being replaced continuously. Delaying in getting them means missing them for good. The pace is such that he who postpones or procrastinates in his gratification is a loser. The race is on, and everyone takes the shortest and quickest route to achieve their objectives by hook or by crook. Not surprisingly, advanced credit, competition, conflict, conspiracy, confrontation, and even criminal behaviour have occurred. Short-term interest prevails. Lifestyle, instead of being a by-product of what one can afford, becomes the end-product to have at all costs. As a result, the success of economic pursuit is the benchmark to replace all human values and relationships. There is no more altruism or higher calling.

The Customer is Always Right

The emphasis that the customer is always right is misleading, as well as a source of stress and mental health problems to those who serve on the front line. What it really means is that the customer has or will have money that we want him/her to spend on our goods and services now or in the future. So, if he/she does not buy today, it is hoped that he/she will buy tomorrow and keep coming back to do so. Thus, this statement should honestly be: money is always right, provided it is not illegally derived. To insist that the customer is always right is more or less to say that there is no personality dysfunction or difficulty, as understood in psychiatry, or persons with negative social traits.

There is another context where clients or consumers, particularly users of government services, are also always right. In this case, it is not directly related to economic performance. The cause and cost of a complaint may affect the outcome of political elections. Thus, complaints, whether reasonable or unreasonable, are feared by both the honest and the corrupt governments. Now, it is further complicated by the manipulation of social media.

The Amoeba and the Specialised Cell

The amoeba is a lowly unicellular organism, but it is free and independent. It moves, seeks food, grows and reproduces itself. Life goes on in monotonous cycles. Only a multicellular organism is capable of a higher quality of life.

The more complex the differentiation and organisation of cells into tissues, organs and systems, the more developed and versatile is the total organism. However, the individual cell must sacrifice its independence and mobility for a specific function. The specialised cell then serves a greater purpose for the benefit of the whole organism.

However, now and then, some cells decide to go their own way regardless of consequences. They proliferate autonomously, spreading from organ to organ and are, in fact, cancerous. Eventually, they harm or kill the host body and themselves. (It is therefore important to detect cancer early and treat it radically.) A man thus has the dilemma of preserving his individuality and independence like the amoeba or fulfilling a prescribed social role like the specialised cell. Stress arises when these two interests are in conflict.

The Soloist and the Orchestra

The aim of many musicians is to be able to perform as soloists. However, the music made by the soloist cannot be compared with that of the orchestra in grandeur, richness and impact. To make great symphonic music, every player, from the first violin to the percussionist, must play his part accordingly and follow the direction of the conductor. Every instrument, note and pause has a specific place. There is no such thing as outplaying one another in loudness or speed or reaching a compromise. Competition exists but only to determine the better player who can lead each section to bring the performance to the highest plane possible. In concertos, the star player is the soloist, and he is accompanied by the whole orchestra. The conductor controls the orchestral players to coordinate with the soloist. They will play as one to create the desired music.

The music that each orchestra can perform depends on its size and component players. To perform well, the orchestra needs time to practise and rehearse. Frequent changes of programmes, musical scores or conductors will affect its performance. To have good music, we also need the necessary support, environment and atmosphere.

Inclusiveness and Exclusiveness

People are always more important than systems because the human element is always crucial. Life is a relationship. It is the relationship between cells that forms tissue, between tissues that form an organ, between organs that form a system, and between systems that form the complete organism.

The highest form of relationship is non-self-seeking love, a love that is inclusive, which grows and makes whole. It is not technical, intellectual or professional, but it enlarges its circle of relationship between persons, families, neighbourhoods, communities and nations. Opposing it is exclusiveness, which is set apart and stands apart from the rest in the cause of perhaps efficiency and excellence. Being distinct, it discriminates, divides, dominates and demoralises. The in-group, however, fosters identity, comradeship and loyalty. If it could be more inclusive instead of being totally exclusive, then its growth and strength would know no boundary. **The secret of successful management lies in the in-group that is inclusive**. Through sharing and belonging, it inspires solidarity that puts the common and higher good first.

Vision and Mission

It is fashionable, if not mandatory, for every institution or organisation to have a vision and a mission statement. And so, many heads will meet for hours and days to draft, re-draft, craft, and re-craft these statements that become the ends themselves, mostly on paper. Implementation is either neglected or compromised. It is not unlike the section leader of each instrument coming together to compose the perfect symphony that is beyond the incomplete orchestra to perform, while the audience is starving for some music to be played.

Policy and Traffic Lights

Policy is like the traffic lights. During the "green wave", the traffic flows smoothly. But when it turns red suddenly, there might be an accident. Then, when it changes to green again, the traffic in front will begin to move, and the queue behind will follow slowly. Thus, after the 2011 Singapore general election, a "new normal" came about. The people at the top quickly responded more openly and inclusively. However, the middle rung reacted tardily, and the lower end hardly moved. If the lights change erratically, there will be traffic jams and chaos.

Helicopter View and Submarine View

Much emphasis has been given to the importance of possessing a helicopter view. The helicopter view sees far and wide and what is on the surface, but to see in depth what is below the surface, the submarine view is needed. There is an earlier saying that people who live in an ivory tower are out of touch with reality on the ground, or they merely act as messengers with misinformation.

The Means and the Ends

It has been said by Søren Kierkegaard: "The end does not justify the means for the means is an end itself". Presumably, even if the end is something good.

A human solution to problems is always at the expense of something else. Every solution creates a new problem. A price is paid by someone, somewhere, sometime. When we cure disease and promote health, we increase life spans and face an ageing population. When we develop our economy and create wealth, we also create pollution and waste. The name of the game is "progress and prosperity". So, to develop, we must create wealth, but to create more wealth, we must create waste through environmental destruction to compete for consumers. Our standard of living is measured by the amount of junk mail in the letter box and reuseable disposables in the garbage bin.

There are two sides to every virtue or vice, depending on the circumstance and perspective. To put it in another way, what is virtue in one context may be a vice in another, and vice versa. It is important to observe rules and regulations, but sometimes, it is more important to bend them. (Although rules should be rules and exceptions should remain exceptions.) A staff member who works overtime may be diligent but may also cause inconvenience to others and incur a higher cost. Perfectionism can be an asset or a setback. As the saying goes, what is meat to one may be poison to another. Furthermore, what is meat today may be poison tomorrow, and vice versa. There is a Chinese saying that the wheel of fortune turns round and round.

The Square One Theory

There is a saying that too many cooks spoil the broth.

To solve the "problem", a team of chief cook, assistant cooks and kitchen hands is formed.

Thereafter, the team meets regularly to discuss the menu and recipe.

Members are also sent for courses and training.

With high expectations, more and more new menus and recipes are created.

Eventually, a glossy cookbook is produced and accepted.

However, the broth is still not served.

Because the cooks are no more cooking and there are no ingredients in the pantry.

Evolution of Knowledge

When we are young, we see only grey.

As we grow and learn, we distinguish black and white.

On becoming adults, we realise the shades of grey in between.

Then, there are experts who can detect black in white and white in black.

There are also others who argue that black is white, and white is black.

Of course, there will be a few who decide what is black and what is white.

In the end it is all grey again.

There is no limit to human intelligence and rationalisation.

Schizophrenic Statistics and Knowledge

As knowledge increases and what has been untreatable in the past becomes treatable, there is also a trend of changing the threshold in criteria and disease definition. As a result, a high percentage of the population would end up suffering from every disease or disorder known. If one were to add up all the percentages or rates of each physical disease or mental disorder published, then everyone would have to suffer from more than one illness. There would be no healthy individuals left, and everyone would end up taking medicines and health supplements.

On the other hand, there are 24 hours in the day. Physiologically, the body needs regular meals, exercise or recreation, and an average of 6–8 hours of sleep and rest to stay healthy and function well. However, full-time jobs nowadays may require the individual to work up to 12–14 hours a day or 60–80 hours a week with no regular breaks for meals. Doctors on duty are expected to be on their feet more than 24 hours at a stretch, 2–3 times a week and not fumble at work. In addition, they are urged to exercise regularly, date and marry, have children and raise them well, be filial to the parents, do voluntary work, and be involved in nation building during the remaining hours of the day. To accomplish all these, more than 24 hours a day would be needed. However, it is argued that people who prioritise, manage their time and do quality stuff would still be able to find time to play golf, attend concerts and go for holidays.

Monkey See, Monkey Do

There is a global culture of colonisation and cloning through international trade and IT. And so, from the monkeys of "see no evil, hear no evil, speak no evil", people have become "monkeys see, monkeys do". They learn to assert and sell themselves, shamelessly or smartly at times. To succeed, there seems to be no place for honesty, humility and modesty. They also adopt the same language and expression, including spelling; the same terminology and titles; the same management and operation; the same franchise and lifestyle; the same idol and icon; the same diet and drink; and develop the same diseases and disorders, etc.

When people sing "Count on me, Singapore" in celebration each year, they also leave behind heaps of affluent litter as "one nation, one people" for others, who are far away from their homes, to clean up their mess. Perhaps there is no alternative or choice in this "monkey see, monkey do" business. It has frequently been repeated that people are too dependent on those in authority. The probable truth is that these people have been too conditioned to obey instructions and follow directions in the mould of "monkey see, monkey do". Some "monkeys" keep setting new benchmarks and gold standards or re-labelling them for the rest with strained resources to chase and copy, often blindly, or for the wrong reasons. Sadly, there is just no catching up. The standard bearers or trend setters will always stay ahead.

"Monkey see, monkey do" also applies to following the footsteps of uncompromising advocates of democracy, human rights, freedom of speech, and capitalism that divides the world between extremism and perhaps introduces a new warfare of "state sans border".

There is also a new breed of monkeys that does not see, does not hear and does not speak.

Change, Choice and Control

Change is a fact of life. And so it is.

Change, such as the growth and development of a child and the four seasons, is part of nature.

They may be anticipated with a welcome. Natural disasters like earthquakes, floods, hurricanes and epidemic diseases are obviously destructive, traumatic and feared, but there are also man-made changes that may be accidental, arbitrary, incidental or intentional, such as industrial disasters, wars, terrorism, economic crises or political upheavals.

Change may be a challenge to conquer and control or a scourge to submit to and survive.

When faced with change, a response is expected. The response may be to avoid, ignore, adjust or adapt to it. There is a choice, although effort is required. When change is threatening, and the effort to cope is exhausting, stress is felt. Such changes are usually imposed on the individual without choice.

There may be arm-twisting, blackmailing or trading off involved.

Successful management of change presupposes choice and control. At a higher plane, it implies the power of politics, the strength of forces, and the reserve of wealth. The developed and powerful, in order to perpetuate control, introduce constant changes, such as IT, the knowledge-based economy, new policies, tariffs, re-structuring, merging, and recruitment of fresh personnel or talents.

Others become stressed because they are at the mercy of imposed changes, which they must keep catching up with to survive.

Id, Change and Virtual Reality

In this era of globalisation, colonisation, cloning and hegemony, there is a relentless emphasis on "change", and so there is an abundance of cliché statements on "change", e.g., "change is the only certainty in life" or "the only constant in life is change". It is strange that in the midst of constant and continuous change, human nature has not changed. (This is evidenced in the proliferation of rules and regulations, protocols and procedures, and law and ethics to control and curb the complex and ingenious human commissions and omissions.)

Nevertheless, the need to change can be a matter of survival for the individual or the society. So, people must be flexible and nimble, innovative, and entrepreneurial. On the other hand, there is also change for the sake of change, which becomes an end in itself. So, people in place must introduce continuous change to appear creative and progressive. Process supersedes the product, and results are inconsequential. In fact, it is difficult to assess or evaluate the outcome of such a change because, before the dust of change settles, another sweeper will come along. While high-flying sweeping is commended, the people on the ground must keep on inhaling the dust stirred up and getting choked. When accounting and accountability are demanded, the virtual reality of "Enron Success" or "WorldCom Connection" could be projected; rhetorical statements and white lies are employed.

Losses in red become gains in black overnight through merging, restructuring, retrenchment and selling off assets.

Virtual reality can also be seen in packaging, advertisements and labels, restructuring and ISOs, JCI, SOPs on paper, measurement and manipulated statistics, relationships in name, title inflation, a free market, future trading and paper assets, etc. In the essence of rapid change, the vision and mission statements of yesterday differ from their translation and implementation today.

There is a saying about "word of honour" in Chinese, which is: "What is uttered cannot be retrieved by the speedy horses". In the modern context of change, it seems that what is uttered disappears into thin air.

One possible explanation for change and the power of change is the insatiable greed or need of the human id for immediate gratification and constant stimulation. Our forefathers, from their experience and wisdom, knew the id well. They cultivated the "superego" through upbringing, only to repress it and emphasise the education of the "ego" to suppress it. Modern entrepreneurs also know the id well, and they stoke it with fad, fashion and fancy for commercial profits or economic gains.

Surrounded by all these changes, we need to strike an active balance of opposite virtues. We must not forget our vocational link to our patients when in pursuit of our career advancement or market forces.

Courtesy, Civic Mindedness, Social Grace and Happiness

There are different perceptions on the regional or global ranking of courtesy, civic mindedness, social grace and happiness. When a high rank is the result of spontaneous and genuine efforts, it reflects good mental health and a cultivated lifestyle, but if it is achieved under duress, then mental health is likely to be at risk.

There could be several possible reasons for a low rank. The emphasis on "no free lunch" or "no one owes you a living" means that "everyone is on his own and for himself" or "I owe no one anything". This would be the root of "kiasuism", which has been overused on almost everything and really means self-centredness and selfishness. Then, there is the elitist top-down modelling effect, where superiority is endorsed, rank is right, money is king, title is queen and bottom up for the unselected is a futile struggle. The gap between the top 20 per cent and the lower 20 per cent widens. On the other hand, a low rank is the outcome and expression of displaced resentment/anger or the ventilation of frustration or plain "bochap-ness" ("who cares"). There is also the habit of complaining against the backdrop of excellence and success being constantly proclaimed. Complaint is safer than criticism. It is all a form of coping with stress in life, and people with no say are saying "no". Finally, there are the "uneducated", antisocial and mentally unwell groups who exist in every society.

Certification, Branding and Franchise

Certification, branding and franchise are big money-making businesses today.

Without certification in areas of education, skill, performance and product, one is handicapped in life.

Entrepreneurs, therefore, create and innovate ways and means of certifying others with qualifications and standards that are marketable.

Life becomes a continuous pursuit of certification and recertification.

Many pay handsomely and willingly to be certified to enhance their market value.

Others have no choice but to submit to the stressful process.

Indeed, not all certifications guarantee quality and delivery.

Only birth certificates and death certificates for all are not earned.

But they, too, could be forged and used for different purposes.

Peddling Stress Management

In medicine, diagnosis is preferably made according to aetiology

Treatment is then directed at the removal of the cause to allow natural healing.

When the cause is not understood or cannot be cured or controlled

Then treatment is symptomatic, or management is palliative.

Modern stress management that earns big money is mostly symptomatic in approach.

There is little attention paid to the cause or stressor.

Often, the stressor is the management that creates unproductive stress.

(see "'Sloggers' and 'Shirkers'" and "History of Corporate Stress")

Stress management should, therefore, target both the stressed as well as the stressor.

Sadly, the peddler is often a helpless victim himself dishing out standard clichés.

Strange Outcome

Despite the crusading and championing of human rights and democracy, it has not produced an equal and egalitarian society.

Instead, the gap between the rich and the poor and the haves and the have-nots has widened.

Such is the power of the predatory globalised/oligarchic corporate organisations, the engine of relentless competition and stress.

Then, there are politically correct denial of differences in individual capability, capacity and caprice that require differential, judicious and enlightened approaches instead of one size fits all.

The Mystery of Logic

To achieve a quality of life that includes a better wage package, there must be significant economic growth.

To achieve sustainable economic growth, there has to be continuous restructuring, upgrading of skills and increasing productivity.

The price for the quality of life is, therefore, relentless change, adaptation and stress.

However, upgrading of skills and increased productivity.

This does not appear to apply to CEOs and directors of MNCs.

The culture and operation of conglomerations is such that the CEOs and directors are paid millions as an entitlement, even when the corporation is not making or losing money.

The lifestyle of entitlement seems to extend to the newer generation, whose bread and butter are provided for by the labour of the older generation.

Having the basic needs satisfied, they are no longer hungry to do any job.

Preoccupation with a hedonistic pursuit replaces the drive to learn and improve.

The id culture of constant stimulation and immediate gratification

Supersedes the Super-ego culture of conscience and ideal.

Meanwhile, the Ego culture struggles to balance them with reality.

Needs, Wants, Technology and Business

Human needs of "yi, shi, zhu, xing, 衣,食,住,行" are basic.

When "clothes, food, dwelling, mobility" are satisfied,

Fashionable clothing, gourmets and beverages, mansion living, automobiles and jets are created.

These new wants become new needs.

Thereafter, needs and wants become intertwined in a continuous response.

Technology is developed to be the answer and provider for constant stimulation and gratification.

Technology is neutral by itself and good for progress and advancement.

However, the hidden "intent" of competitive interest, business profit, and control of the market keeps spiralling in changes.

Products in satisfactory usage are constantly phased out by the withdrawal of services and spare parts.

New products are tweaked here and there as progress and are desirable.

In the process, earthly resources are exploited, wastes are created, and environments are destroyed by consumerism and materialism.

Man becomes stressed to learn, unlearn and relearn to deliver.

The misfits, unfits and unwilling people become unemployable and redundant because not all persons have the same capabilities and abilities.

But man likes to think or believe he has rights, freedom and choice.

In reality, he is also a slave to needs, wants and business greed.

The population is not only ageing, but the number of misfits, unfits (and "unwilling") is also growing.

They feel deprived, frustrated, angry and resentful.

Mental and physical health become an issue and a burden.

Technology creates new jobs but also destroys old jobs.

Restructuring of the economy and upgrading of skills have become a necessity

Meanwhile, partial solutions are found in foreign talents or workforces and the invention of computers, machines and robots.

Approach to Problems

What is the problem? (It is obvious that the problem must be identified.)

Whose problem is it? (Responsibility or liability is implied.)

Why is it a problem? (Question of circumstance or context.)

How to deal with the problem? (It depends on individual orientation.)

Orientation to the Problem

Philosophy:	Altruism, ideal, pragmatism
Point of View:	User, provider, purchaser, payer, politician
Purpose:	Objective, goal
Priority:	Urgency, agenda, resources, viewpoint again!
Professional:	Expertise, training, practice, territory
Progress:	Not synonymous with new and change, or technology
Politics:	To ensure continuation of power or popularity
Policy:	Subject to political, economic, social forces
Payment:	Funding, reserves, profits
Partnership:	To enhance image and competition
Propaganda:	Mechanism to achieve covert/overt set goals
Prosecution:	Medico-legal implication, litigation, insurance

The different orientations to dealing with problems are not mutually exclusive. There is much overlapping, interplay and compromise.

Punitive or Therapeutic Approach to Medico-legal Issues

In the past, the sentencing of convicted offenders was restricted to the issue of whether they were of sound or unsound mind. The disposal was limited. However, there has been a better appreciation of the grey areas of those who are intellectually challenged or mentally disordered in terms of their responsibilities. The approach now is more humane and therapeutic.

Generally speaking, depending on the stage of development, value system and the availability of resources, society may **medicalise** some deviant or anti-social behaviours and treat them, or **criminalise** such behaviours, and punish the individuals responsible. Thus, drug problems, for instance, may come under the Ministry of Home Affairs or the Ministry of Health or both in different countries.

Healthy Environment, Healthy People

Someone has said that there is **no healthy person without a healthy environment** (and perhaps vice versa). So, there are movements and organisations, such as the United Nations, promoting Healthy Person-Healthy Environment projects and programmes. These would include:

Physical — Good housing and transport, clean air and water, supply of food and energy, a hygienic environment, sewage and sanitation, control of pests and diseases, etc.
Social — Opportunity for education, fulfilling employment, fair income, religious freedom, racial harmony, law and order, justice, individual rights, space for recreation, a healthy lifestyle, etc.
Psychological — Security, safety, a stable and caring society, satisfying relationships at home, work and play, etc.

These factors play important parts in both physical and mental health and are often taken for granted.

Therefore, a clinical multidisciplinary team has an important role and functions.

The government or society that provides a healthy environment and promotes healthy persons deserves as much credit (if not more) as the physician.

Nature, Meaning / Concept of Stigma

The meaning and concept of stigma includes a sense of shame, disgrace, disdain, derision, discrimination, blemish, contempt, condemnation, etc.

The Origin of Stigma

The origin of stigma would include a sense of being superior and righteous, prejudice, ignorance, misconception or misunderstanding, fear of the unknown, uncertainty and unpredictability.

The Subjects or Contexts of Stigma

Stigma has existed since ancient times. It is present in many cultures and situations and for many individuals in varying degrees, from mild and subtle to strong and obvious. It may occur in different primitive and underdeveloped societies or ethnic groups with different social classes and castes. It may also be due to cultural and religious customs and taboos. For instance, in the past, stigma was experienced for those who were not married when above a certain age or in mixed marriages, being an unwed mother or born out of wedlock, being divorced or committing adultery. In religion, it may refer to others who are considered or looked down on as being ignorant and superstitious. In lifestyle and occupation, it may apply to poverty, prostitutes or sex workers, menial and lowly jobs, unemployment, illegal activities, prisoners, ex-convicts, etc.

In the medical context, it is well known for applying to sufferers of mental disorders or medical illnesses. It is common, though lesser now, to involve sexual gender dysphoria or orientation, patients with sexually transmitted diseases, HIV/AIDS, cancers, dementia, intellectual disabilities or mental retardation, disfigurement, a past history of leprosy or tuberculosis, which could even extend to personnel looking after them.

Core issue — due to "**Not knowing how to relate to the other person**".

The core issue of stigma in mental illness/disorders appears to be that of "**not knowing how to relate to the other person**" due to ignorance, fear, a lack of exposure and contact, or misconceived influence from others. This is particularly true of sufferers with **psychosis**, where there is a **breakdown** in **conformity** of appearance and behaviour **with** the **community**; a **breakdown** in **communication and interpersonal relations** because of incoherent or irrational and irrelevant thought and speech of the patient; and a **breakdown** in **control** when the **individual** acts out his psychic or psychotic experience in a frightening and threatening manner that cannot be understood or predicted. As a result, there is uneasiness or discomfort and the fear of being at a loss on what to do and how to respond to this person, which leads to the avoidance of contact and relation.

Thus, stigma occurs when there is a breakdown in conformity (with the community), communication (interpersonally) and control (of the individual). Relationships become distant and alienated, discriminated or even condemned.

Due to ignorance, misconception, prejudice and misgivings (or fear of the unknown), uncertainty, and unpredictability, this stigma is **extended to other mental disorders**, such as anxiety, depression and obsessive-compulsive symptoms, which are **common** and **prevalent** and may affect **anyone**. Stigma perpetuates in a vicious circle when symptoms are concealed, consultation is avoided, or treatment is non-compliant, but when one is well-informed of the nature of matters and has been trained, engaged and experienced in managing or understanding these symptoms, then that is when stigmatising wears away.

There is a saying that "**familiarity breeds contempt**". It is actually unenlightened familiarity that breeds stigma and snubbing. **Enlightened** familiarity breeds acceptance and accommodation. Families and mental health professionals show that relationships can develop, and stigma can be reduced. "Sufferers" could lead by example to demonstrate that recovery and reintegration are possible.

Comparison of Mental Disorders and Medical Disabilities

The physically disabled are viewed with great sympathy, and understandably so; for example, there is a code-based reading and writing system like Braille for the blind and sign language and speech therapy for the deaf and mute; there are many voluntary organisations and lobby groups to advance their rights and interests; and jobs are created or reserved for them. Other aids include specially modified cars and reserved parking lots, wheelchairs, ramps, lifts in buildings and user-friendly toilets, public transport with special facilities, easy access to places of interest, etc. However, those who are mentally disabled are still avoided, ignored or even rejected. People do not expect the blind to see, the deaf to hear, and the paraplegic to walk normally, and so they bend backwards to help and accommodate them, even inventing robots and prostheses to rehabilitate them. But the public and sometimes our own rehabilitation programmes expect, if not demand, that they behave and function like ordinary people. However, some of these individuals with severe volitional and cognitive impairment are like a "psychic tetraplegic", or a computer that hangs. Indiscrimination over enthusiasm could, therefore, be stressful and counterproductive.

The **consequence of stigma** in mental illness/disorders leads to cover-ups, secrecy, avoidance, alienation, discrimination, non-compliance in treatment, and suffering, with negative outcomes of a loss in productivity and dependency.

Management

Continual proper education, appropriate exposure/engagement/experiences, and sustained campaigns for the public and volunteers are necessary. There must also be "enlightened familiarity" to relate with human compassion, acceptance and accommodation.

Strategic Goals to Target

Subjective perceptions: With understanding, acceptance/accommodation, support, compassion, hope.

Objective perspective: Public campaigns/education, social reforms/destigmatisation, medical research/treatment, improved prognosis/hope, economic opportunities, political legislation.

Promoting Mental Health

Someone has said that there is **no healthy person** (whether physical, psychological and social) **without a healthy environment** (whether physical, psychological and social). There is an active balance between the healthy person and a healthy environment.

Apart from mental disorders of known biological/organic causes, the **majority** of mental disorders can be said to be **induced**

by stress or stressors in life. There are predisposed **intrinsic** factors of individual vulnerabilities and **extrinsic** factors of environmental pressures.

Common symptoms of mental disorders are anxiety and depression.

So far, mental health programmes and strategies **focus** mainly on the suffering or the casualty.

Management emphasises early detection and early treatment, such as coping with stress, providing hotlines, community and welfare services, medications, psychotherapy, and lifestyle changes.

If **prevention is better than cure,** then there should also be a **focus** on or recognition of an **unhealthy environment**, which is often the **causative** factor or stressor. Stress management ought to involve **employers** (including the managers, executives, supervisors, etc.), the **government** and policy enforcement, and **public** perception and attitude.

With a preoccupation on **economic growth**, there is a constant emphasis on competition, restructuring, upgrading of skills, increased productivity, and added consumerism and materialism. Granted that stress is unavoidable to ensure survival, it is not always necessary. There needs to be a shift in paradigm on the responsibility of the environment (in its management) to reduce **unnecessary stress** due to selfishness, greed and incompetence, so as to reduce mental health problems. It takes insight and effort to achieve an active balance.

Early Detection and Assessment of Mental Health

Any prolonged change, disturbance or loss in one's Five Appetites and one Mc PIE (a mnemonic for depression) should be reported over time regarding one's state of health.

Five Appetites

1. **Sleep** — *too little, too much, interrupted, insomnia (Causes: anxiety, depression, psychotic symptoms)*
2. **Eating** — *anorexia, bulimia, paranoid avoidance, obsessional rituals*
3. **Work** — *function, performance and productivity*
4. **Relationship** — *sexual, social and family interactions*
5. **Recreation** — *exercise, habits (e.g., alcohol, drugs, gaming, etc.), hobbies*

Loss of one Mc PIE (in depression)

1. ***M**emory*
2. ***C**oncentration*
3. ***P**leasure*
4. ***I**nterest and*
5. ***E**nergy*

Ecc. 1:9,11

What has been will be again.
What has been done will be done again.
There is nothing new under the sun.
There is no remembrance of men of old.
And even those who are yet to come.
Will not be remembered by those who follow.

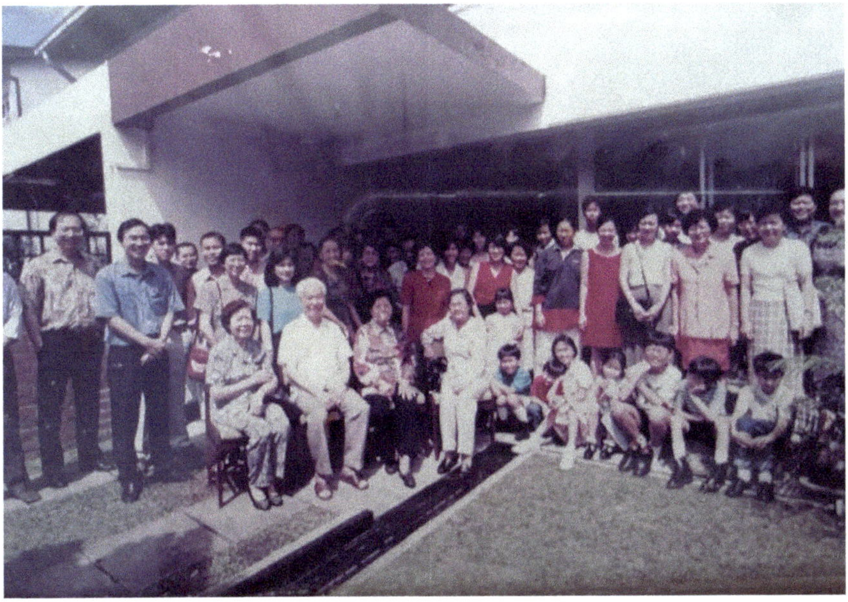

Figure 1. The Chee clan at a Chinese New Year gathering with my father, who was the patriarch of the extended family.

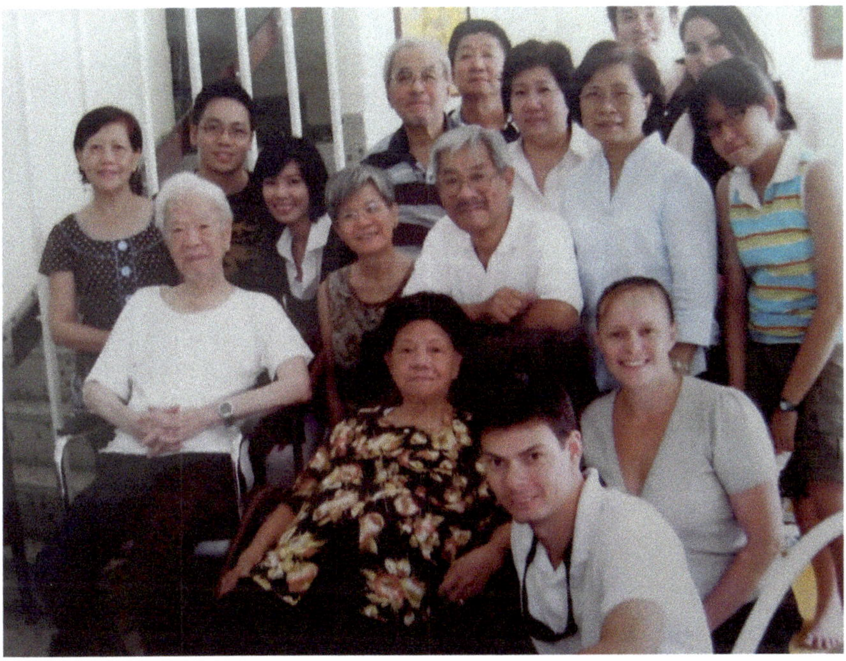

Figure 2. My parents and siblings with their children.

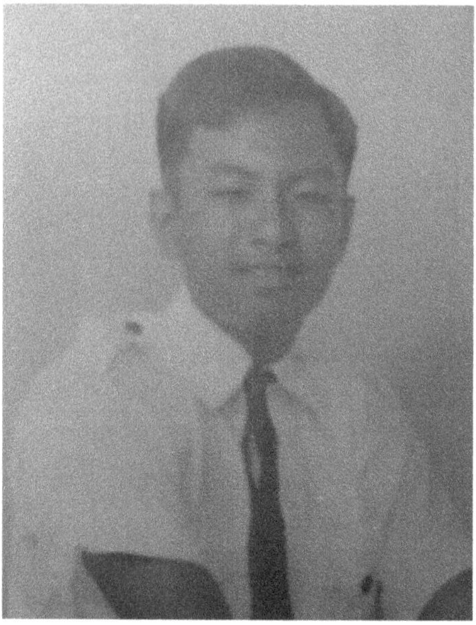

Figure 3. Here, I am a student wearing the Chinese High School uniform.

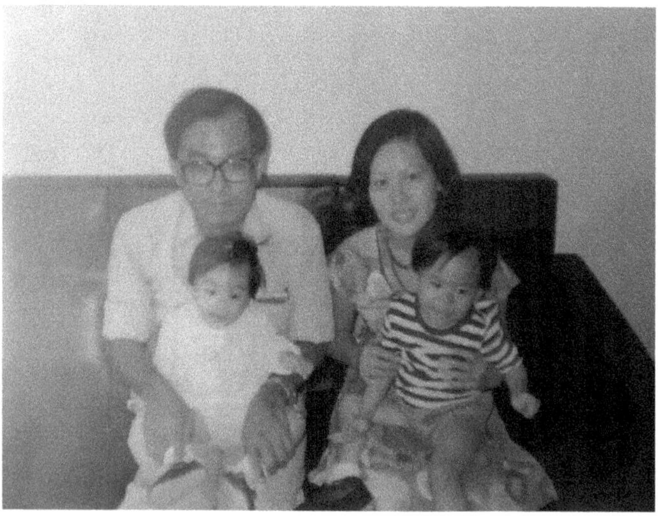

Figure 4. Family photograph when our children, Yung En and Sung Ping, were young.

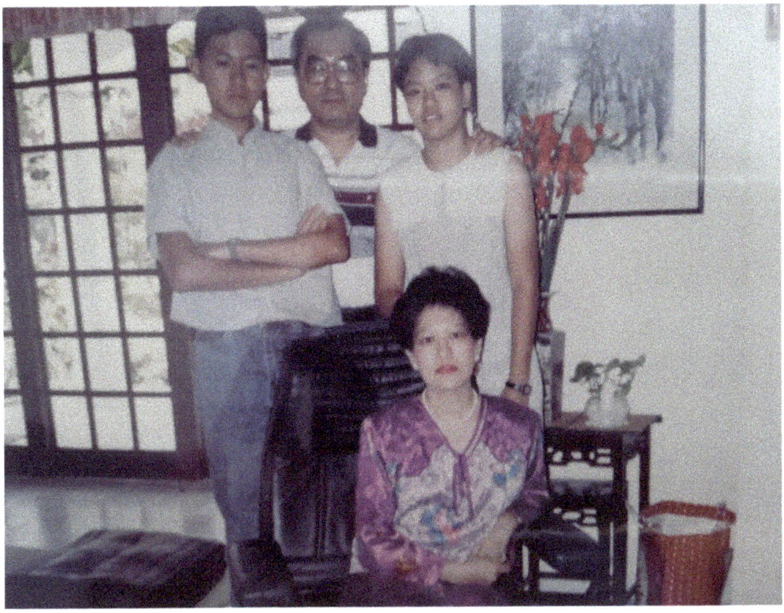

Figure 5. Another family photograph, this time with our children as teenagers.

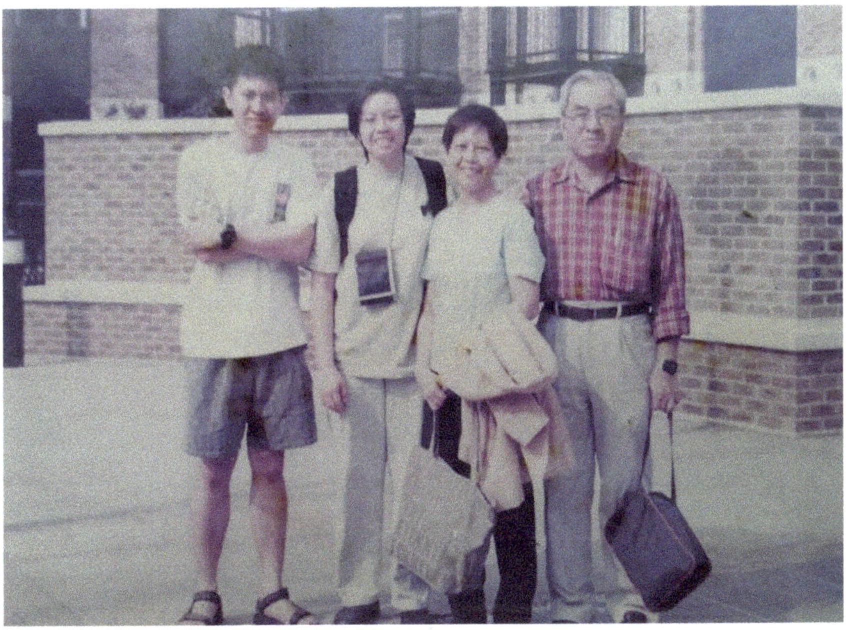

Figure 6. Family photograph in front of our London apartment when Sung Ping was in medical school.

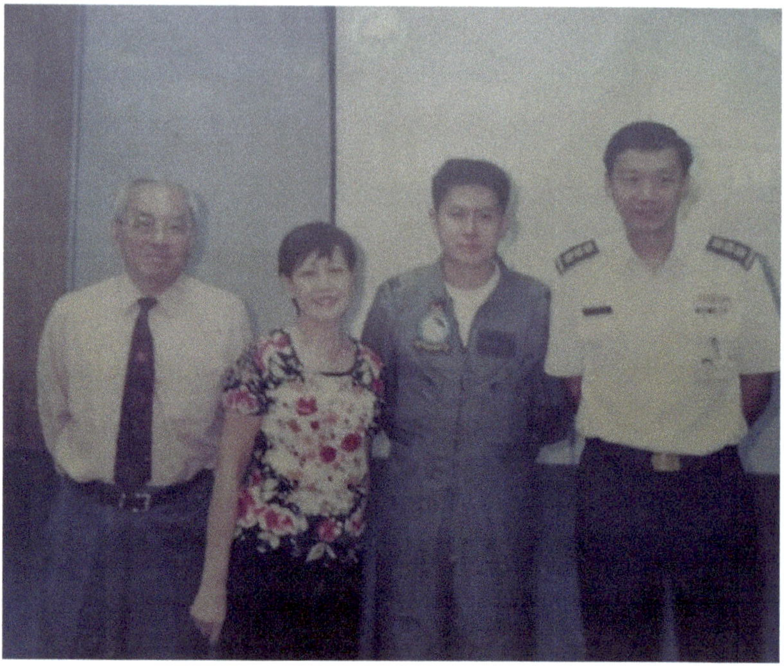

Figure 7. Sung Ping with his chief after qualifying as a RSAF pilot.

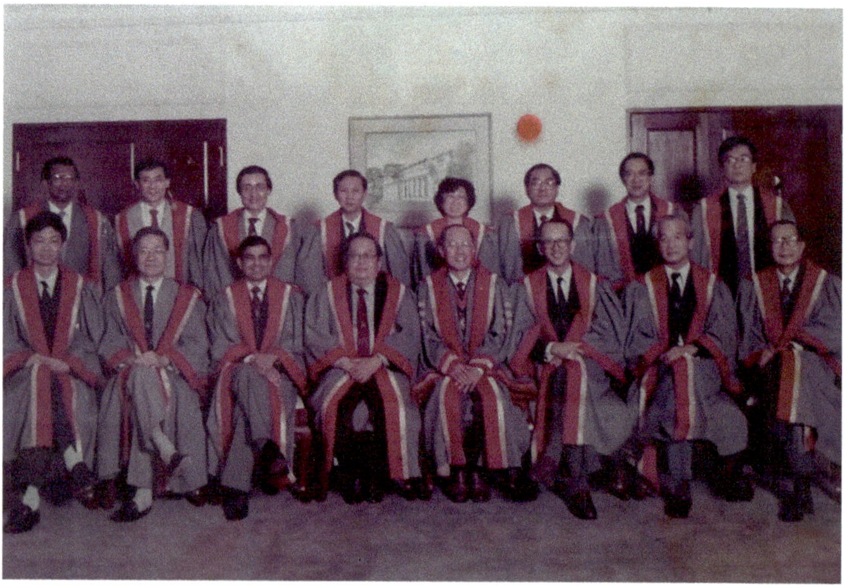

Figure 8. Academy of Medicine Chapters of Specialists Chairpersons.

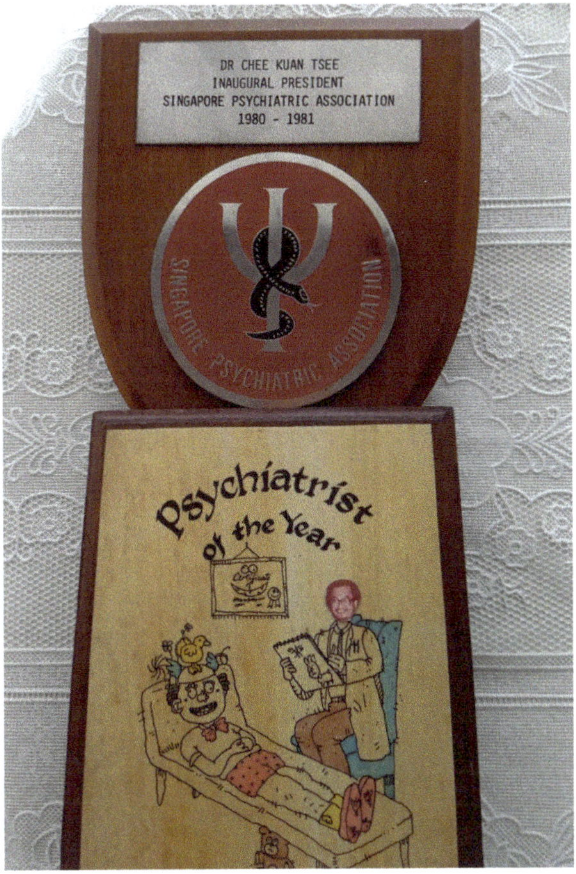
DR CHEE KUAN TSEE
INAUGURAL PRESIDENT
SINGAPORE PSYCHIATRIC ASSOCIATION
1980 - 1981
SINGAPORE PSYCHIATRIC ASSOCIATION
Psychiatrist of the Year

Figure 9. Top plaque: Inaugural President of Singapore Psychiatric Association; lower plaque: light-hearted honour from my children.

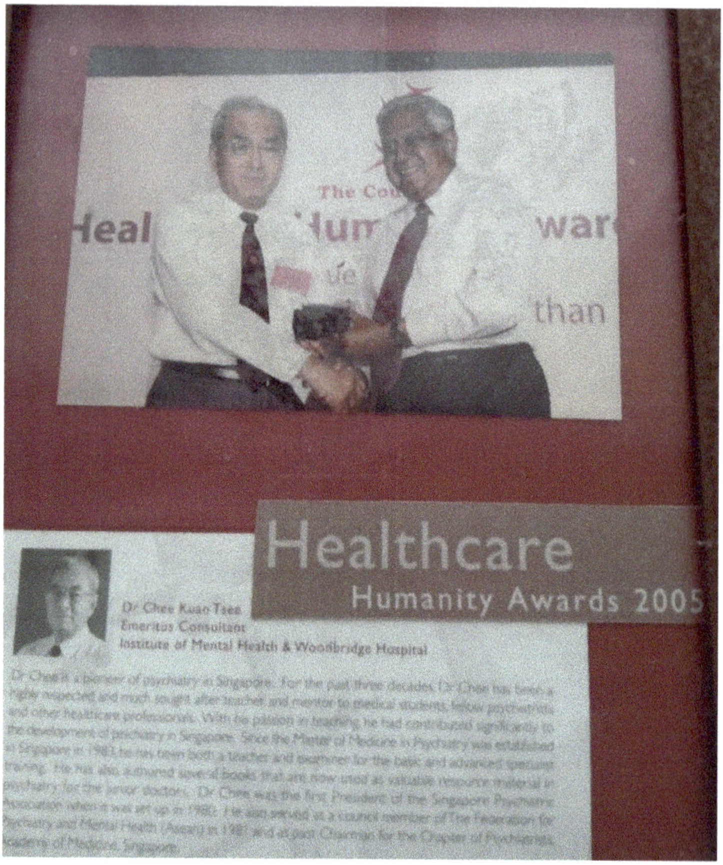

Figure 10. Receiving the Healthcare Humanity Award from the late and former President S. R. Nathan.

www.ingramcontent.com/pod-product-compliance
Lightning Source LLC
LaVergne TN
LVHW051054210926
848486LV00002B/110
9789819832866